Calisthenics:

Core

Crush

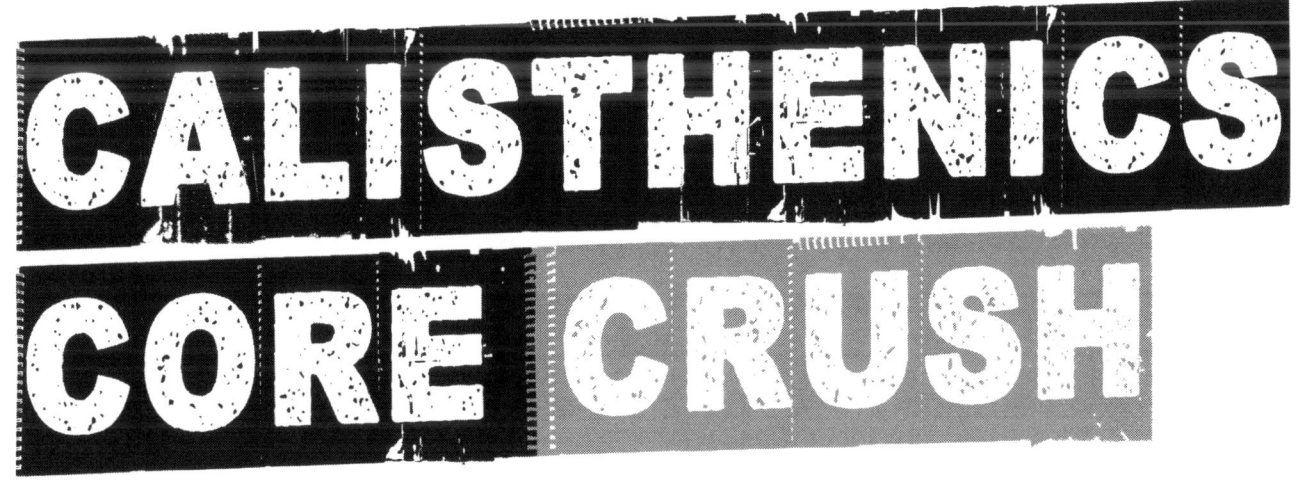

THE #1 SIX PACK ABS BODYWEIGHT TRAINING GUIDE

PURECALISTHENICS

Copyright © 2016

Pure Calisthenics

All rights reserved. No part of this publication may be reproduced, distributed, or transmitted in any form or by any means, including photocopying, recording, or other electronic or mechanical methods, without the prior written permission and consent of the publisher, except in the case of brief quotations embodied in product reviews and certain other non-commercial uses permitted by copyright law.

Disclaimer:

This guide has been created for informational and reference purposes only. The author, publisher and other affiliated parties cannot be held in any way accountable for any personal injuries or damage allegedly resulting from the information contained herein, or from any misuse of such guidance. Although strict measures have been taken to provide accurate information, the parties involved with the creation and publication of this guide take no responsibility for any issues that may arise from alleged discrepancies contained herein. It is strongly recommended that you consult a physician, personal trainer and nutritionist prior to commencing this or any other workout or diet plan. This guide is not a substitute for professional personal guidance from a qualified medical professional. If you feel pain or discomfort at any point during the exercises contained herein, cease the activity immediately and seek medical guidance. This resource has been created to teach calisthenics in a progressive way, and you should not advance until you have completed the simpler exercises as recommended with perfect form. It is strongly recommended that you use a spotter or personal trainer at all times.

calisthenics

[kal-*uh* s-**then**-iks]

Noun

1. *Gymnastic exercises designed to develop physical strength, vigor and grace of movement, usually performed with little or no special apparatus.*

Origin

Greek *kallos* "beauty" + *sthenos* "strength" + -ics.

BEFORE YOU BEGIN:

BONUS GIFT: FREE CALISTHENICS TRAINING PROGRAM

As a token of gratitude for picking up this book we'd love to give you a free body-weight exercise program to help you on your way to superhuman shape!

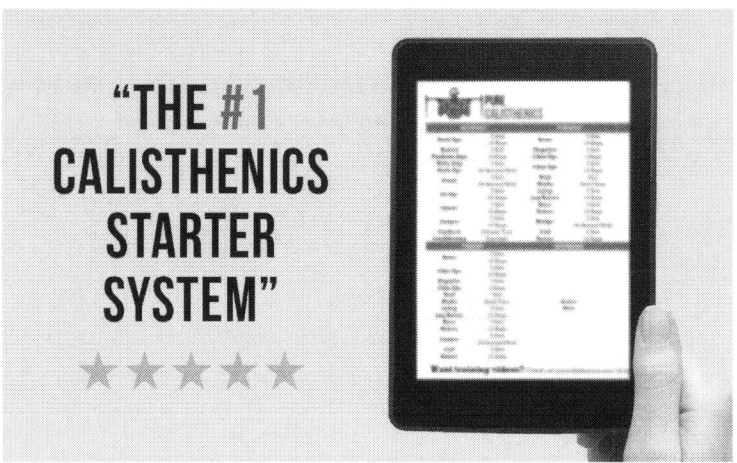

Visit **www.purecalisthenics.com** for your training program!

Contents

Before you Begin: 6
Introduction 11
How to Use This Book 13
    1. Prepare 13
    2. Focus 13
    3. Commit 13
    4. Think Long-Term 13

1. What is Calisthenics? 15
    How Does it Work? 15
    What Does it Do? 15
    Who is it For? 16
    How Can I Get Started? 16

2. Diet and Nutrition 19
    Hydrate 19
    Eat Right 19
    Eat for Your goal 20

3. Know Your Body 23

4. Warm-Up & Preparation 27
    Hands 28
    Cardiovascular 28
  Mobility / Motion 29
    Upper Body 30
        Wrist Rotates 31
        Shoulder Rotates 32
        Shoulder Dislocates 33
        Scapula Push-Up 34
        Scapula Pull-Up 35
        Scapula Dip 36
    Core 37
        Hip Rotates 38
        Side Leans 39
    Lower Body 40
        Open / Close Gates 41
        Deep Squat 42
        Mountain Climbers 43
        Frog Hops 44

Flexibility & Stretching 45
Upper Body 46
- Wrists & Forearms 47
- Chest & Shoulders 48
- Chest II 49
- Upper Back 50

Core 51
- Side Stretch 52
- Cobra 53
- Cat 54

Lower Body 55
- Calves 56
- Hamstrings 57
- Groin 58
- Glutes 59
- Hip Flexor 60
- Hips II 61
- Quadriceps 62

5. Exercises **65**
Core 66
Fundamentals 67
- Sit-Up 68
- Crunch 70
- Plank 72
- Side Plank 73
- Extended Plank 74
- Bicycle Kicks 75
- Elbow to Knee Cross 76
- Russian Twists 77
- Dish Hold 78
- V-Up 79
- Lying Leg Raises 80
- Rear Arch 82
- Rear Support 83
- Knee Raises 84
- Leg Raises 86
- Window Wipers 88

Dragon Flag 91
- Candlestick Position 92
- Tuck Dragon Flag 94

>> Single-Leg Extension Dragon Flag 96
>> Negative Dragon Flag 98
>> Complete Dragon Flag 100
>> Dragon Flag Kicks. 102
> Half Lever. 105
>> Tuck Half Lever 106
>> Partial Half Lever 107
>> Complete Half Lever 108
>> Half Lever Leg Extensions 110
>> Half Lever Single Leg Extensions 112

6. Cardio & Conditioning 117

> Interval Sprints 118
> Skipping 119
> Jumping Squat 120
> Squat Thrust. 122
> Mountain Climbers 124
> Jumping Lunge. 126
> Star Jumps 127
> Burpees 128
> Advanced Burpees 130
> Bear Crawls 132
> Other 133

7. Progressing With Calisthenics. 135

8. BONUS: Free Training Program 137

> Like This Book?. 138

INTRODUCTION

Congratulations, you have just invested in the world's most effective training system. This book is part of The SUPERHUMAN Series, and in this edition you will be chiseling out a popping six-pack and obliques fit for a GREEK GOD!

This guide has been designed to teach calisthenics in a progressive way, with multiple variations on popular exercises increasing in intensity and difficulty as you make your way through. Follow our guidance to the letter, adhere to the structure set out and you will experience MIND-BLOWING results.

Whether you are completely new to exercise or switching over to calisthenics from weightlifting or anything else, this book is for you. Get started now and take the first step on the path to a stronger, fitter, more powerful you.

To stay up to date with the latest trends in bodyweight exercise, please join us online at purecalisthenics.com for training tips, equipment reviews, nutrition advice and more. You can also find us on Twitter and Facebook - just search 'Pure Calisthenics'.

For more calisthenics resources, check out our full range of books by searching 'Pure Calisthenics' on Amazon. For now, it's time to get down to business. Read on, comrade, and unlock your potential with Core CRUSH!

Train hard!

The Pure Calisthenics Team

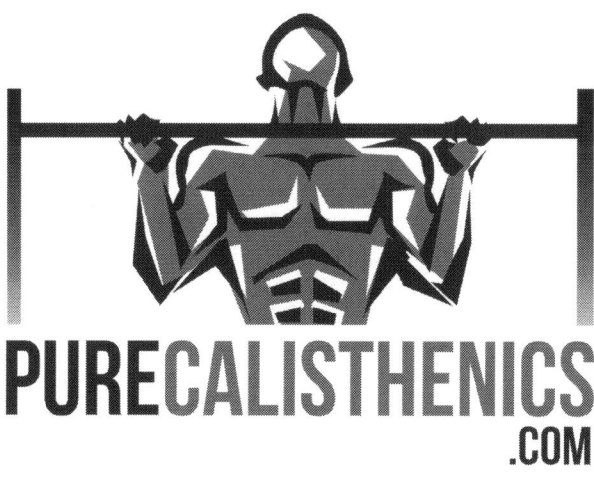

How to Use This Book

This book is your training bible. You should not merely read the words; you should LIVE by them. Yes, there will be times when you want to give up, but pressing on ahead is what separates the best from the rest.

Use these 4 quick tips to help maximize your results:

1. Prepare
Don't just dive straight into the exercises headfirst and go crazy, you will put yourself at risk of injury. Read through the introductory chapters of this book so you know exactly how to approach your training.

2. Focus
Calisthenics is not just about physical strength, but also mental fortitude. Your friends may swear by free weights and there's nothing wrong with that if they want to train isolated muscle groups. You, however, are training to achieve complete body perfection and you must stand by your decision. Don't allow anyone to influence your thinking – you are training for YOUR goals, not theirs.

3. Commit
As with any form of exercise, you need to be fully committed to a consistent workout program if you want to see results. Don't think you can simply throw in a few body-weight movements here and there and go home looking like a Greek god. Calisthenics requires you to GIVE everything if you want to TAKE everything. Follow a proper training schedule and stick to it. You'll find a link to our free program at the back of this book.

4. Think Long-Term
Following on from the above, it is important to maintain a long-term vision for your training. There is no miracle formula for a better body, but calisthenics is as close as you can get. Set realistic goals and commit to achieving them within a reasonable time frame and, in time, you will achieve incredible levels of strength and physical ability. Don't forget to keep track of your progress and celebrate the little wins along the way.

Now the pep talk is out of the way, let's move on!

1. What is Calisthenics?

If you're reading this book then the chances are you've already looked into calisthenics, probably read a few articles online and watched some videos of seemingly superhuman feats of strength by famous practitioners on YouTube.

These guys have it all; traps that reach up to their ears, sculpted shoulders, bulging chests, forearms like Popeye, abs you could grate cheese on and legs that could propel them to the moon. And all without pumping iron? Well, pretty much.

How Does it Work?

Calisthenics, by definition, is a form of exercise that consists of various gross motor movements using your own bodyweight for resistance, normally without equipment or apparatus, with the exception of basic items such as a pull-up bar or parallettes.

This is the art of training your body as nature intended; not by isolating muscle groups and using complex man-made machinery that you would never find out in the real world, but by using the tools you are already equipped with. With calisthenics, your body is your gym, and the world is your playground.

What Does it Do?

Calisthenics is the art of strengthening your entire body as a unit, eliminating each weak link in the chain until every fiber of your being is working in total harmony to produce extraordinary levels of strength.

Training like this achieves results you can use in the real world. Think about it, how often do you need to bicep curl something, or flap cables around over your head in everyday life? These are all man-made inventions designed to make single muscle groups strong IN THE GYM, but as soon as we step outside it becomes somewhat irrelevant.

To perform at maximum capacity in everyday life, or to acquire formidable strength and fitness for your sport, you need to be strong everywhere, not just in certain places.

Calisthenics strengthens every muscle group and every link between those muscle groups. It is the ultimate form of exercise for creating true strength that you can use every day, whether it be for regular tasks, your favorite sport or just showing off!

1. What is Calisthenics?

WHO IS IT FOR?

The simple answer to this question is that calisthenics is for everyone. Practicing bodyweight training can help anyone achieve a stronger, fitter, more flexible body.

Whether you are a lean athlete wanting to pile on more muscle mass, a 200-pound bodybuilder seeking to get shredded, a kick boxer requiring greater range of motion or simply starting up with exercise for the first time, calisthenics is the ultimate solution.

Don't just take our word for it. Professional sports teams and global militias often utilize calisthenics for its explosive effectiveness and practical application. You can use your bodyweight to train any place, any time, making it the benchmark fitness solution for high level operators across the world.

Don't get stuck performing the same old isolated exercises in the gym for years on end, choose calisthenics and take your gym with you wherever you go!

HOW CAN I GET STARTED?

One of the great advantages of calisthenics is that it's super simple to get started. You don't need a gym membership or any prior experience, and you can begin with simple exercises today.

With that in mind, here's a few key tips to make life easier for those just getting started:

1. Use a credible guide: This is your starting point! Don't dive straight in and use guesswork to correct course, as this often ends in disappointment or, worse, injury. Whether you choose to follow this guide or something else, the most important thing is that you stick to it like glue, and let the experts guide you to success.

2. Establish a program: Training without a program is like driving around a strange place without a map. In order to stay on track and keep up to date with your progress, you need a schedule. You can get one at the back of this book, or work with a trainer to create your own.

3. Get a training partner: Tests prove that accountability is a hugely effective catalyst for increasing performance. For us, this means getting a committed training partner and supporting each other on the journey.

Above all, starting up is as simple as putting on your sweats and getting out there. So, step up and step out, companion, it all begins here!

"There are no limits. There are only plateaus, and you must not stay there, you must go beyond them."

Bruce Lee

2. Diet and Nutrition

We can practically hear some of you screaming, 'I know what to eat, just get to the good stuff already!'

Well, we're going to shut you down like a rat-infested restaurant right now because diet and nutrition are the foundation of a great body and it would be a dereliction of duty to neglect this area.

If you want to maximize your results then don't skip this part.

Hydrate

Water is life. We need it to transport vital nutrients around the body and to keep our muscles and minds functioning at full capacity.

Most people simply do not drink enough water day-to-day, which means both their performance *and* their recovery is greatly impaired.

According to The European Food Safety Authority, men should be drinking about 2 liters of water per day while women should get about 1.6 liters. This is, of course, a general guideline but if you are not hitting these figures you may be affected by dehydration. We recommend speaking to a physician or nutritionist to discuss your requirements.

If you are taking a supplement such as creatine, which affects the way that your body processes water, then you will need to drink more. Check out the label on all of your supplements and always ensure you take on board enough fluids.

While we're on the topic, steer clear of alcohol and fizzy drinks if you want to get ripped. They're packed full of carbs and sugar, and won't do you any favors whatsoever.

Eat Right

Your particular goals will determine your diet, but there are some general guidelines to follow here if you want to get in the best shape possible.

Eat clean: We're not asking you to become a hippy or go plucking fruits from trees, but it really pays to cut out processed food and other junk. Check the labels and pick up fresh foods which contain a single ingredient – i.e. whatever it is actually supposed to be – rather than something packed full of preservatives and lord knows what else.

Mix it up: You've heard it said over and over and now you're going to hear it once again; a balanced and varied diet is the key to good health. This means a mixture of proteins, carbohydrates and fats. Check out the following examples for some inspiration:

Proteins: Organic meat, poultry, fish, eggs and dairy are primary sources of protein.

Carbohydrates: Fruits and vegetables are a great source of healthy carbohydrates, as are sweet potatoes, wholegrain pastas, brown rice and similar grains.

Fats: Forget the myth of fat being bad for you. The type found in good quality meats, nuts, seeds, fish and olive oil is an essential part of your daily diet.

EAT FOR YOUR GOAL

When you strip diet and fitness down to their core elements it becomes very simple. If you want to gain weight and muscle mass, you simply have to eat more calories than you burn off.

If you want to maintain your weight and refine your body then you should be aiming to eat around the same amount of calories as you burn off. If you want to cut down then you should be burning off more calories than you are eating.

There are plenty of resources out there to assist you with your particular objective, but we would advise against obsessive calorie counting. Food should be something to look forward to and you will soon start to resent it if preparation becomes a chore. By all means use tools and technology to ensure you are on the right track, but don't beat yourself up over fractions of a gram.

With that said, you should be aware of your macros and make a conscious effort to meet them on a daily basis. If you're not sure what this means, it is essentially just the combination of fats, carbs and proteins which make up your diet. Everybody is different and only you can determine what is appropriate for your body and goals, but if you are unsure, it pays to contact a professional nutritionist for guidance.

Planning meals in advance and cooking in bulk is super useful here, as it cuts out the guesswork and reduces the risk of making poor decisions on impulse!

We could write a whole book on diet and nutrition, and perhaps we will, but this one is about calisthenics, so for now we must move on. Suffice it to say, though, that you should pay special attention to your diet and take the time to investigate it thoroughly in order to maximize your results.

"Looking good and feeling good go hand in hand. If you have a healthy lifestyle, your diet and nutrition are set, and you're working out, you're going to feel good."

Jason Statham

3. Know Your Body

Think you know your body? Think again. It's one thing to isolate muscles with regular exercises such as the bench press or bicep curl but it is entirely another to employ whole groups at the same time to squeeze out that last gut-busting muscle-up or planche.

Putting yourself under such intense strain can be dangerous if you don't know what you are doing, so it is important to familiarize yourself with your body to ensure you are utilizing it correctly and not putting yourself at risk of harm.

We suggest keeping a body map handy. You'll find a basic one on the next page, but it's a good idea to take your learning further, otherwise you may have no idea what we mean when we discuss certain muscle groups.

There is no shortage of quality resources out there when it comes to biomechanics and the study of the human body, and the more you learn the more control you will have over your progress and results.

In addition to DIY textbook style studying, we always recommend hooking up with a qualified and reputable personal trainer or physician to assess your individual needs and goals, since we cannot be there to advise everyone in person.

Super important: If at any time you feel pain or discomfort during exercise, STOP. Try some slow, steady movements to test the area and stretch it out gently.

If pain persists or worsens, call it a day and seek advice on the issue. Refer back to the body map to hone in on the area and speak to a physician for further advice.

Only return to training when you can comfortably perform movements without feeling any pain or impingements. Do not be tempted to 'power through' an injury as this will only exacerbate the issue and delay your recovery time. It is much smarter to take a short break and get back on track quickly than to finish your session at the cost of weeks or even months out of action.

Remember, calisthenics may be completely different to anything you have performed before. You will likely awaken muscles you never even knew existed, and it is probably going to hurt like hell, so make sure you are suitably prepared.

To help brace your body for action we'll be covering warm-up and preparation next.

3. Know Your Body

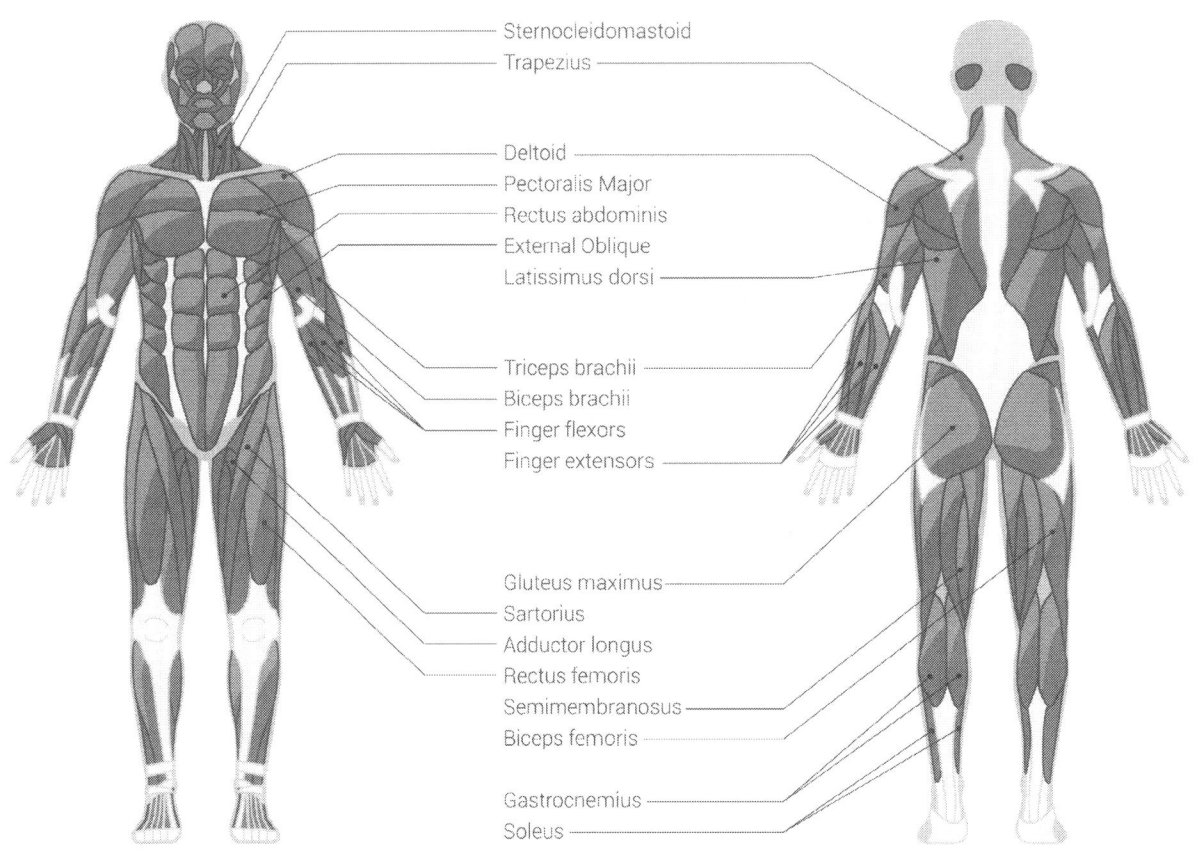

Above: A basic body map showing the major muscle groups. It is possible to drill down into much more detail, but we simply do not have the scope to cover everything in this guide. We highly recommend that you take your learning as far as time allows.

Remember, although we share the same basic physiology - with the exception of the obvious differences between the male and female anatomy - every individual is unique. Genetic factors beyond our control give us the blueprint with which we must work.

Instead of trying to 'fight' your genetics, we recommend working with them in order to sculpt your perfect body. If this sounds a bit heavy, don't worry, it simply means getting to know your strengths and weaknesses and working with those, instead of trying to force yourself down a path your body isn't prepared for.

That's not to say you can't build your dream physique, only that you should take a smart and informed approach. As always, we recommend speaking to a pro for more advice.

"Success is no accident. It is hard work, perseverance, learning, studying, sacrifice and most of all, love of what you are doing or learning to do."

Pele

4. Warm-Up & Preparation

Whether you are a seasoned gym-goer or a complete newbie, calisthenics will shock your body to the core. You will awaken muscles you never even knew existed and aches and pains will spring up all over as you become stronger as a unit. For this reason it is essential to prepare properly if you want to achieve stunning results..

The benefits of warming up are threefold:

1. By getting the blood pumping and warming up your muscles you can hit the ground running and maximize performance during your workout.

2. You minimize the risk of getting injured during training, meaning you won't have to cut sessions short or drop out entirely due to niggles or tears.

3. Stretching helps you become more flexible over time, meaning you can increase your range of motion and subsequently push your body to new limits. As you scale up in this way you will gain unprecedented strength and capability.

Some people consider warming up to be a waste of time, but if you're not willing to put in an extra 5-10 minutes per session then we would have to question your commitment to calisthenics and fitness in the first place.

When you stop thinking of a warm-up as a chore and see the serious value it brings, it will revolutionize your workout and help you along the way to results you never thought were possible. But hey, don't just take our word for it.

Consider any of your favorite sports teams or stars. From professional football clubs to mixed martial artists, Olympic rowers to tennis players and everyone in-between, there is not a single person who steps out without some form of warm-up. If it's good enough for the greatest in the world, it's sure as hell good enough for us.

Remember: This book is focused on calisthenics, and while we can cover some essential mobility and flexibility exercises we simply don't have space for a complete solution. Use the following as a guideline and build your own warm-up routine over time. Add it to your routine and consider it sacred. Don't rush it, and don't skip it.

So, now that you understand the myriad of benefits warm-up and preparation brings to your workouts, let's get to work, shall we?

4. Warm-Up & Preparation

HANDS

In order to transfer maximum power from your hands to whatever piece of apparatus you are using you must ditch the gloves and go bare skin. This may seem somewhat counterintuitive, because many gloves do offer additional exterior grip and most will make things more comfortable. Long-term, though, they will do more harm than good.

Consider pull-ups, for example. The extra layer between your hands and the bar means you are only as strong as your grip on the inside of the gloves. It doesn't matter how sticky the outsides are, because when that inner material starts sliding around, you'll drop like a sack of spuds.

So, the only way to transfer 100% of your energy to the bar is to make a direct and true connection. Your hands are going to take a battering and might feel sore at first but over time you will condition them to cope with these stresses and ultimately reap the rewards of a vice-like grip.

If you are using chalk or liquid chalk to help with your grip you might find your hands become very dry over time. Be sure to wash it off completely once you're finished and, if necessary, use a moisturizer.

You are unlikely to tear your hands apart when you are just getting started, but if for any reason you do cut them open don't act tough and carry on as this could put you out of action for weeks. It's best to rest for a day or two and let them heal before continuing.

Calluses are to be expected, but cuts and scars are not badges of honor to be worn with pride; they are a sign of bone-headed stupidity. Take care of your hands, and they will take care of you!

CARDIOVASCULAR

Once your hand preparation is taken care of, the first port of call in your pre-workout warm-up is to raise your heart rate and get the blood pumping.

Try 5-10 minutes of the following dynamic exercises to achieve this:

• Jogging, skipping, star jumps, cross-trainer, rowing

There are plenty of other ways to get your cardio fix, so mix it up a bit each day. Don't go overboard and leave yourself keeled over in exhaustion, but make sure it is intense enough to leave you a little out of breath. Your heart should be beating faster, and a light sweat is a good sign that you are ready to move on.

Mobility / Motion

You've completed phase one of your warm-up, so the blood should now be pumping around your body, letting you know that you are ready to loosen up the areas you'll be hitting in your workout. We'll now run through some gentle mobility exercises designed to loosen up your limbs and increase your range of motion.

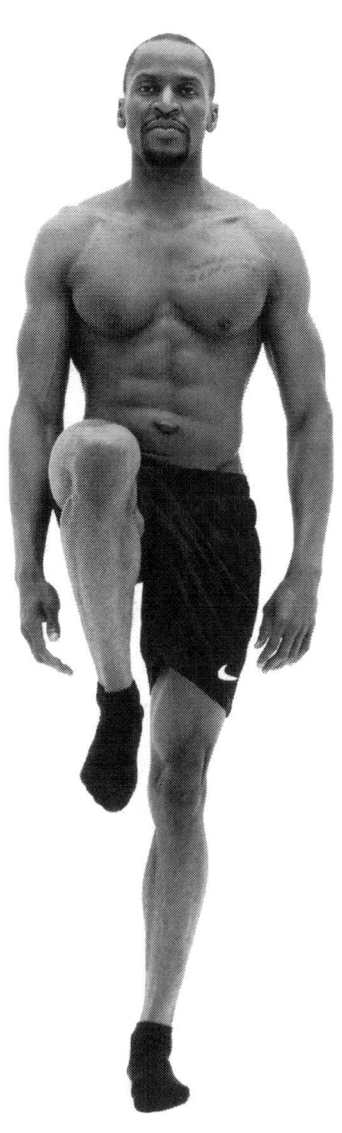

Upper Body

You will use every muscle fiber your upper body has to offer when training calisthenics so it is essential to get it ready for the task. Spend another 5-10 minutes going through the following, paying special attention to the areas of the body you plan to work out.

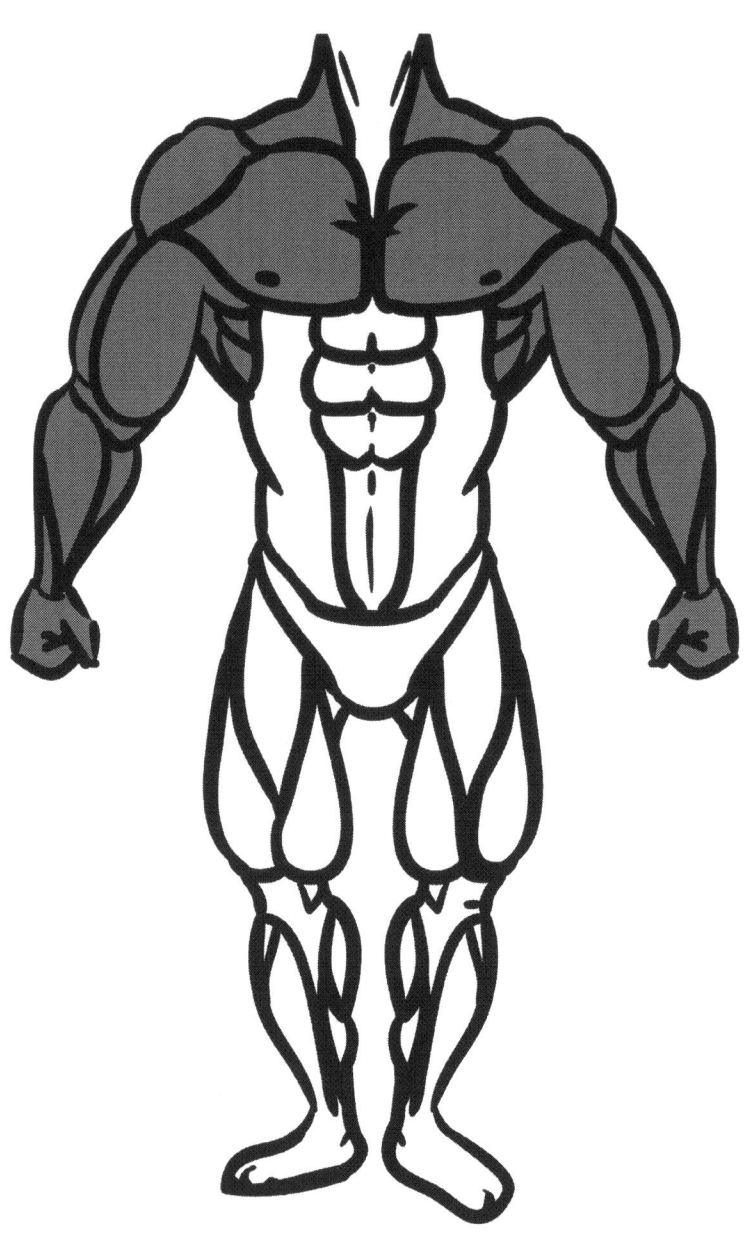

Upper Body

WRIST ROTATES

Your wrists are taxed in almost every calisthenics exercise, so try this simple warm-up to keep them strong and safe.

Perform: 10 seconds in each direction.

1. Extend your arms straight out in front of you.

2. Rotate your wrists clockwise for 10 seconds.

3. Switch directions and go again.

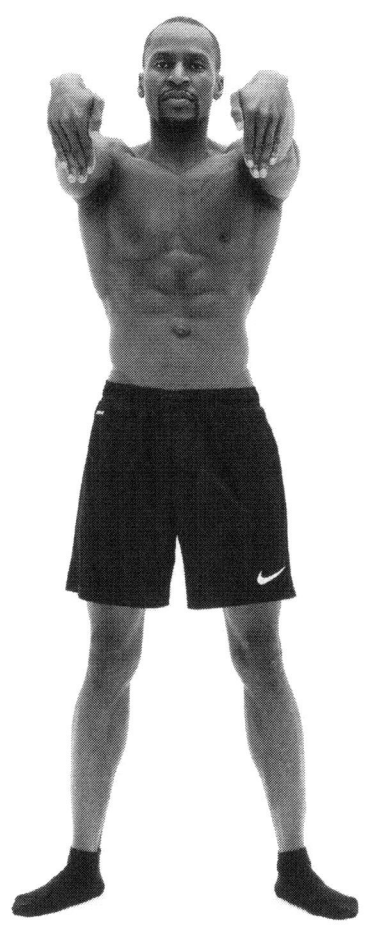 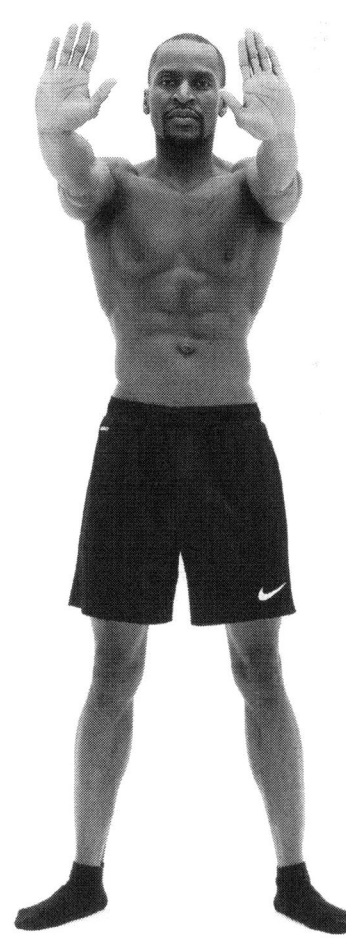

SHOULDER ROTATES

This is a simple but effective warm-up for the rotator cuff and shoulders.

Perform: 10 seconds in each direction.

1. Stand firm and extend both arms straight out to your sides.

2. Rotate arms forwards for 10 seconds.

3. Stop and do the same in reverse.

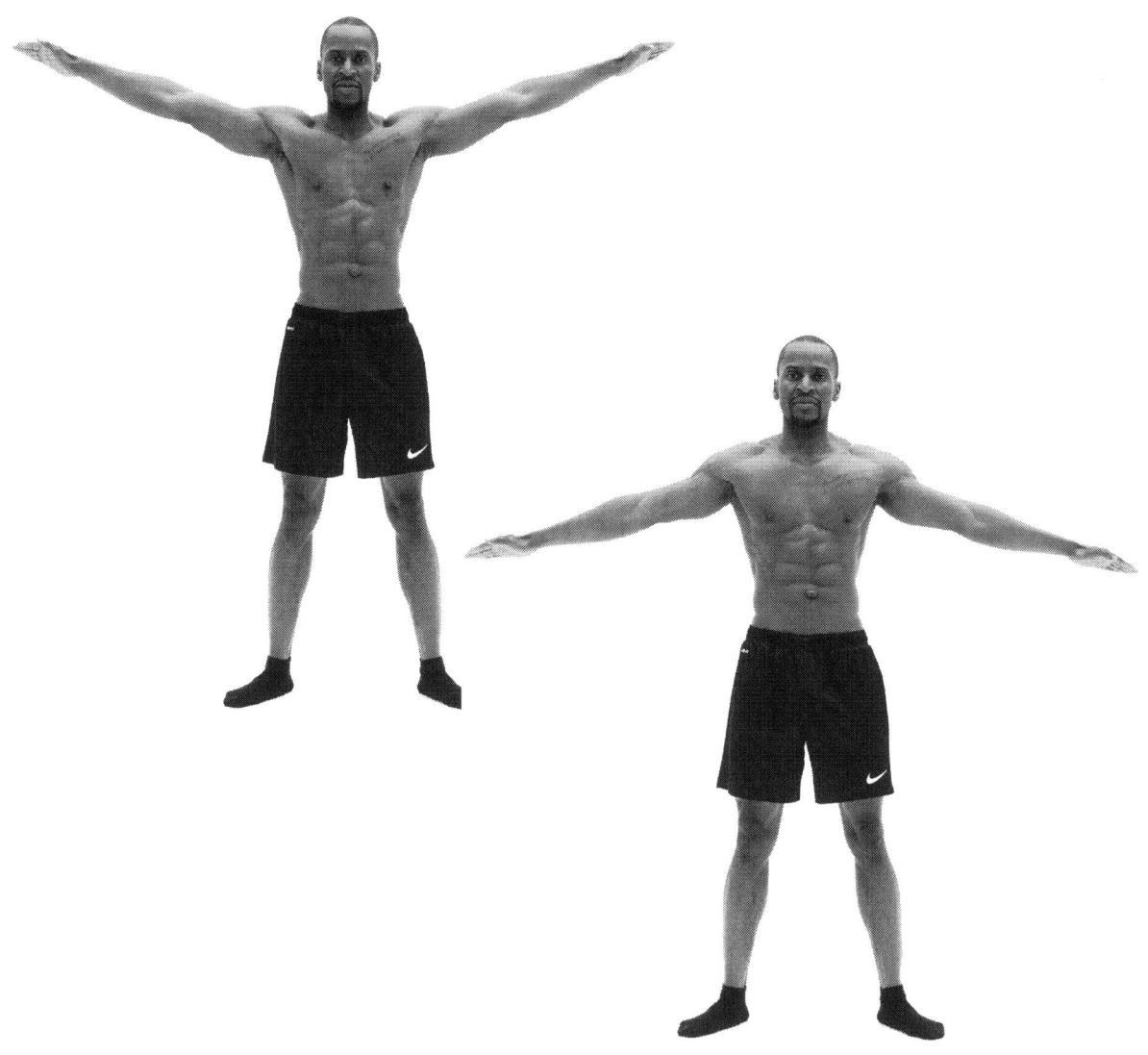

SHOULDER DISLOCATES

Don't panic, the clue isn't actually in the name this time! Your shoulders won't really pop out during this exercise, but they may still be a little uncomfortable at first. Since you will be opening up your shoulders, back, chest and arms here you will probably feel tightness in one or more areas.

Perform: 2 sets of 8 repetitions.

You will need: a long, lightweight bar.

1. Stand up straight, feet shoulder width apart, hands a little wider apart on the bar with an overhand grip (palms down).

2. Lift the bar up directly over your head and in one smooth motion bring it down to rest on your lower back, keeping your elbows locked at all times.

3. Reverse the movement, bringing the bar back to the front of your body to complete one rep.

You may struggle with this at first, so try sliding your hands wider apart along the bar until you find a position that allows you to perform the movement without bending your arms.

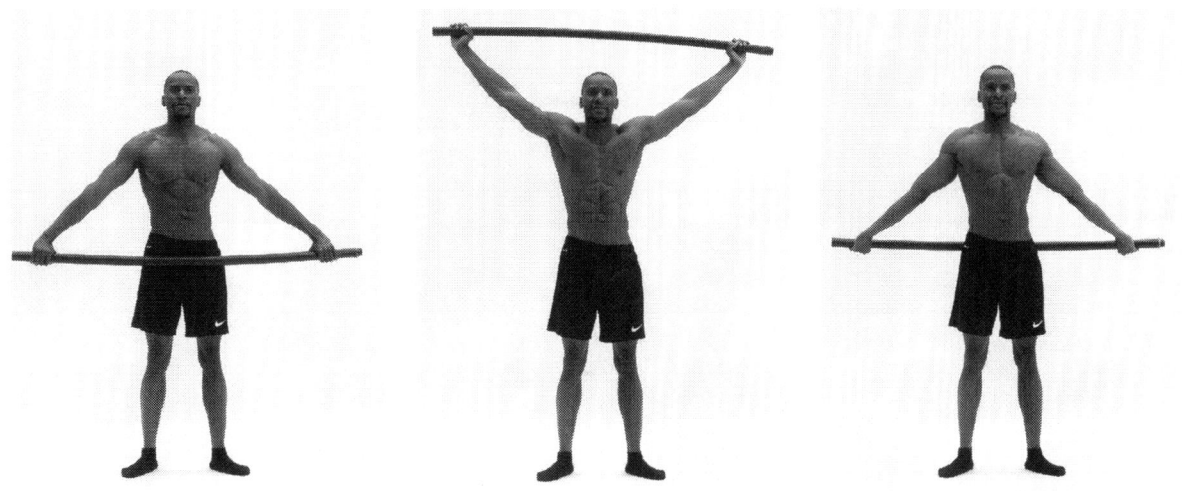

Scapula Push-Up

The scapula push-up is an excellent way to prepare your upper body for a beating. In particular, this will mobilize the muscles in your upper back and shoulders.

Perform: 8-10 repetitions.

1. Get into push-up position (see push-ups if unsure), placing your knees on the floor if you are just starting out.

2. Keeping your elbows locked and arms straight, let your chest sink towards the floor and squeeze your scapulae together at the same time.

3. With your elbows still locked, reverse this movement, lifting your chest back up and separating your scapula so that your back arches and your spine rises.

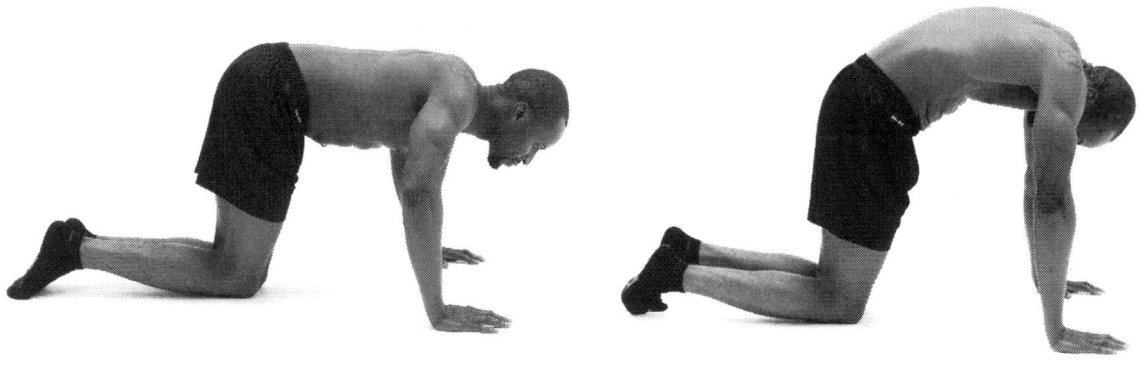

SCAPULA PULL-UP

The clue is in the name again; we'll be working your scapula and upper back here to great effect with an outstanding strengthening mobility exercise.

Perform: 8-10 repetitions.

You will need: a pull-up bar.

1. Grasp the bar overhand and allow yourself to hang with your arms and body totally straight, feet off the floor.

2. Relax, aiming to get your shoulders to touch your ears so your scapulae are elevated.

3. Keeping your arms and elbows locked in position; try to pull your scapulae downward.

4. Hold for 1-2 seconds and then lower back down to the starting position.

The movement involved in this exercise is so subtle that it is best demonstrated with good old-fashioned arrows! You may find this movement very difficult initially, but as with all things your mobility and control will improve over time so stick at it.

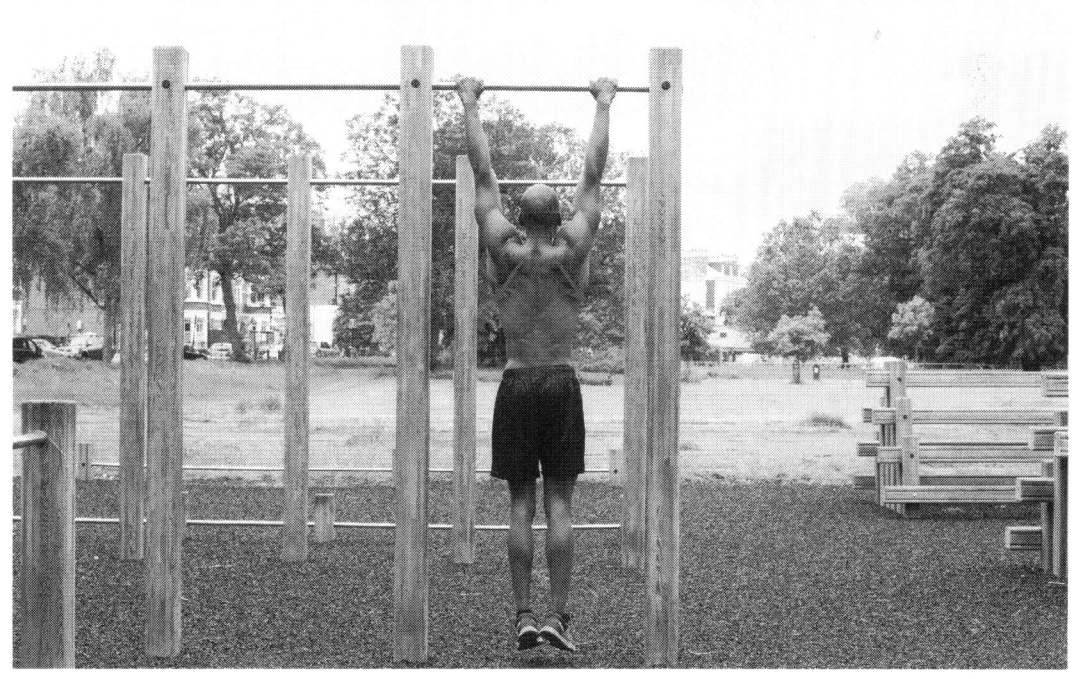

Scapula Dip

This motion will fire up your shoulders and give you greater range of movement for 'pushing' exercises such as, well, push-ups!

Perform: 8-10 repetitions.

You will need: parallel bars or dip station.

1. Grab the bars and lock your elbows, lifting your feet up and supporting your bodyweight in a neutral position.

2. Keeping your elbows locked and arms straight, sink your body down aiming to get your shoulders to meet your ears (or as close as you can).

3. With your arms still locked straight, push back upwards as high as possible, effectively trying to get your shoulders and ears as far apart as you are able.

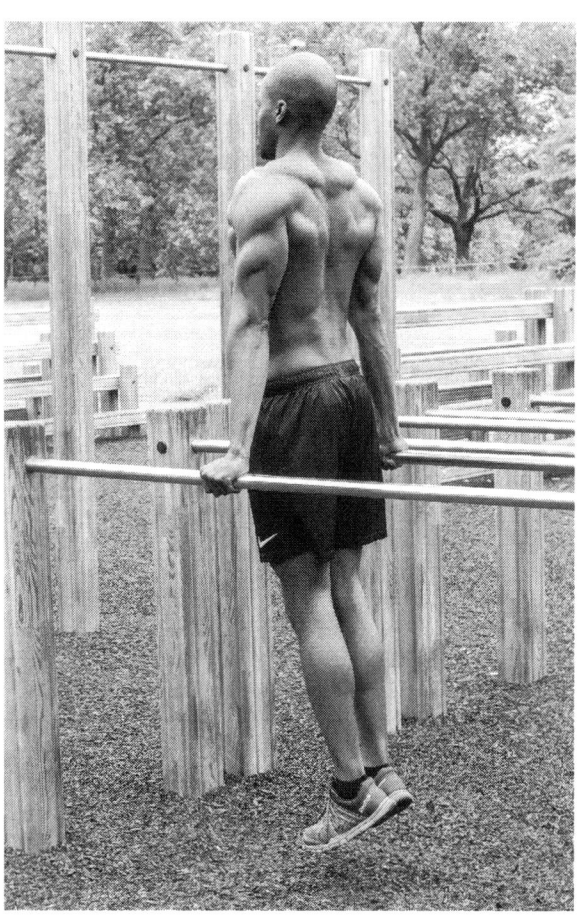 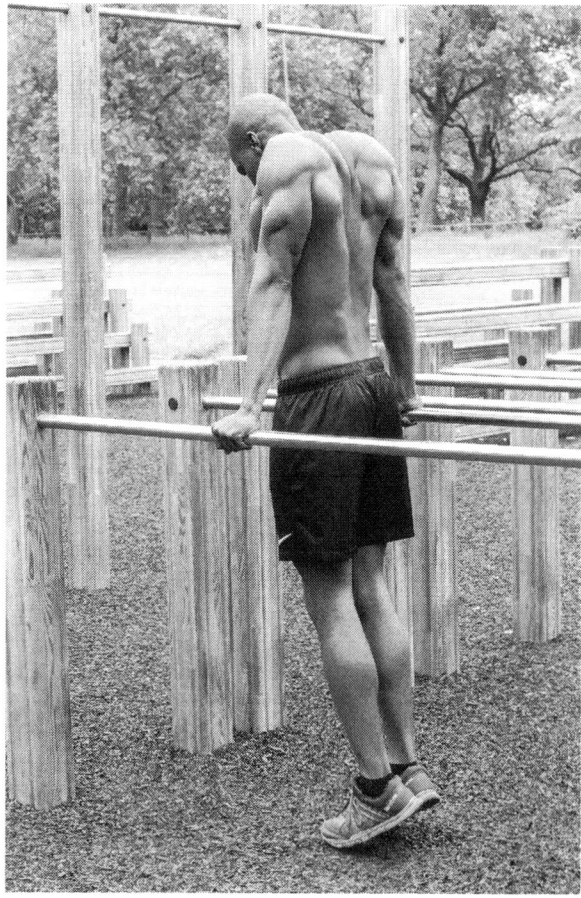

Core

If you are taking your warm-up seriously then you should have broken a sweat by now. You will be glad to know that core mobility is nice and quick to address! Let's get to it.

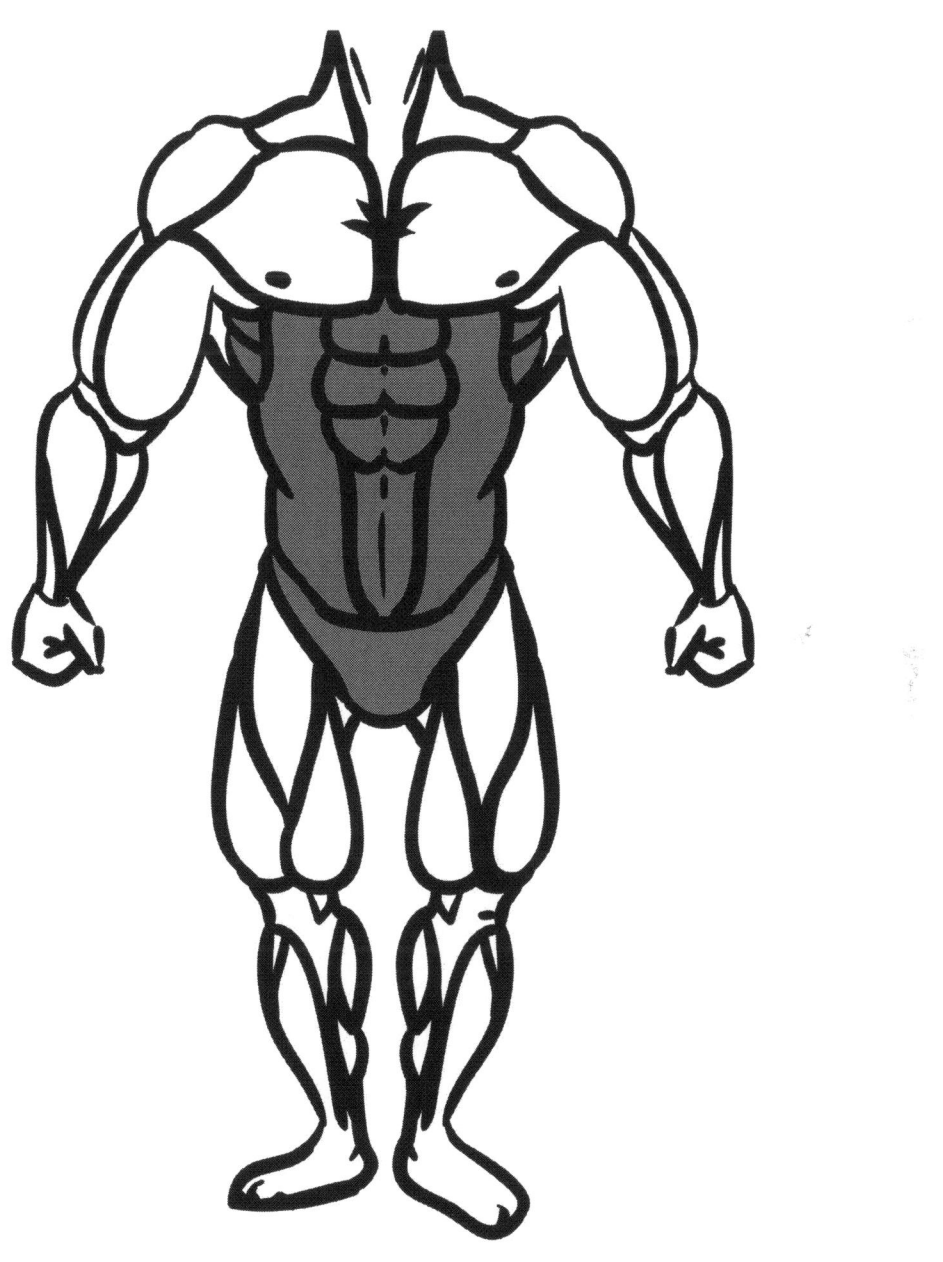

4. Warm-Up & Preparation   -   Mobility / Motion

HIP ROTATES

Get your hula on to open up those hip flexors and increase your range of motion.

Perform: 2 sets of 8 repetitions in each direction.

1. Stand upright and place one hand on each hip.

2. Slowly rotate your hips clockwise in a 'hula' movement, aiming to keep your knees and back neutral, focusing the movement in your hips.

3. Repeat the movement counter-clockwise.

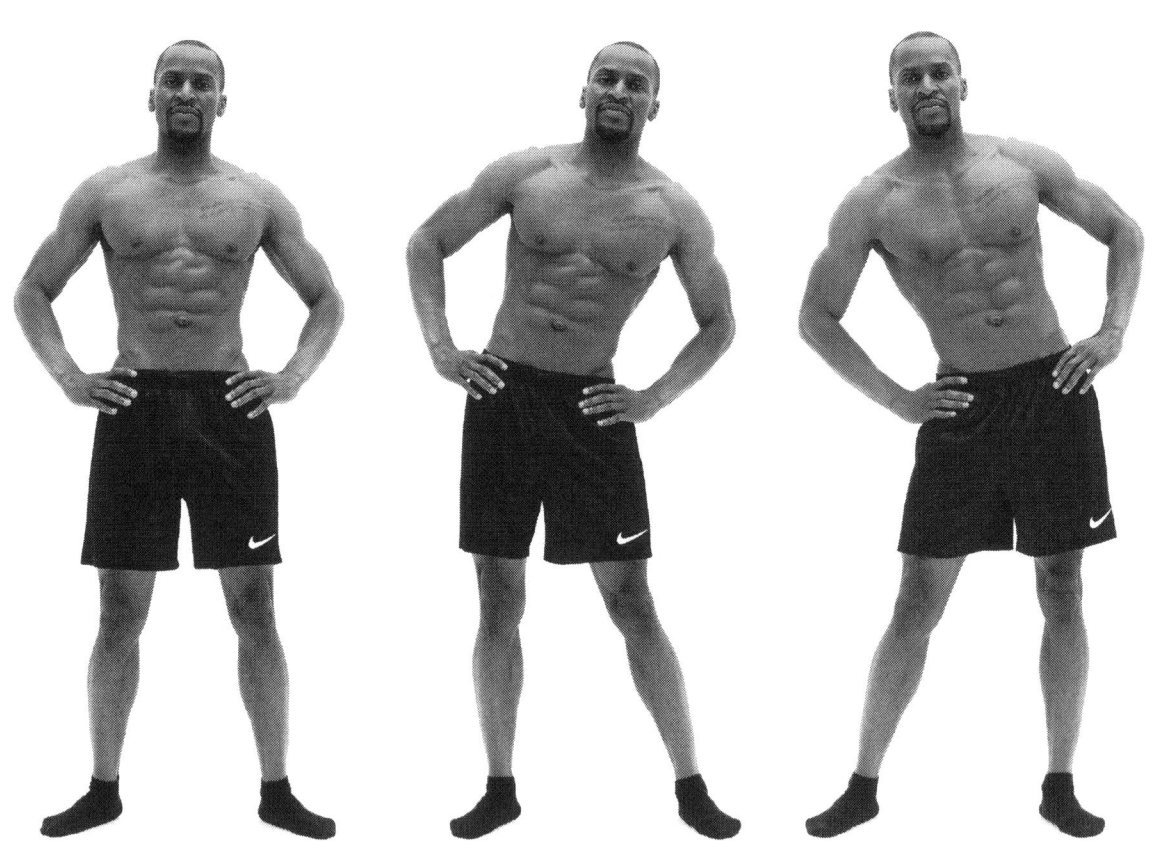

SIDE LEANS

Tight obliques and an inflexible lower spine can greatly inhibit your range of motion, so perform this movement to loosen up these areas.

Perform: 5 repetitions in each direction.

You will need: a long, lightweight bar.

1. Stand upright with your feet just wider than shoulder width apart, grasping the bar over your head.

2. Keeping your arms straight, feet rooted and shoulders in position, lean over to one side to stretch out the other.

3. When you have reached as low as possible, reverse the movement and repeat the exercise on the other side of your body.

Variation: You can perform this exercise without a bar if needs be, simply lean over to one side and grab your leg with the closest hand, bringing the other arm up overhead.

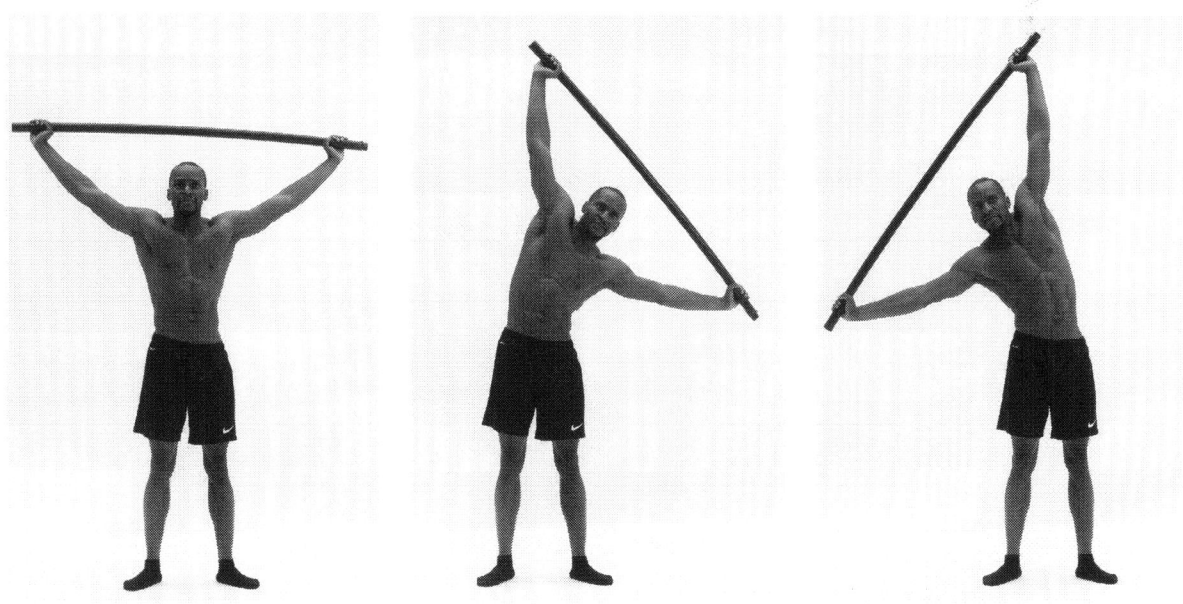

LOWER BODY

Even if you're not training lower body you will still be using it to get around so it's good practice to perform these exercises, too. Check out the following and incorporate them into your routine, or simply practice them on off days.

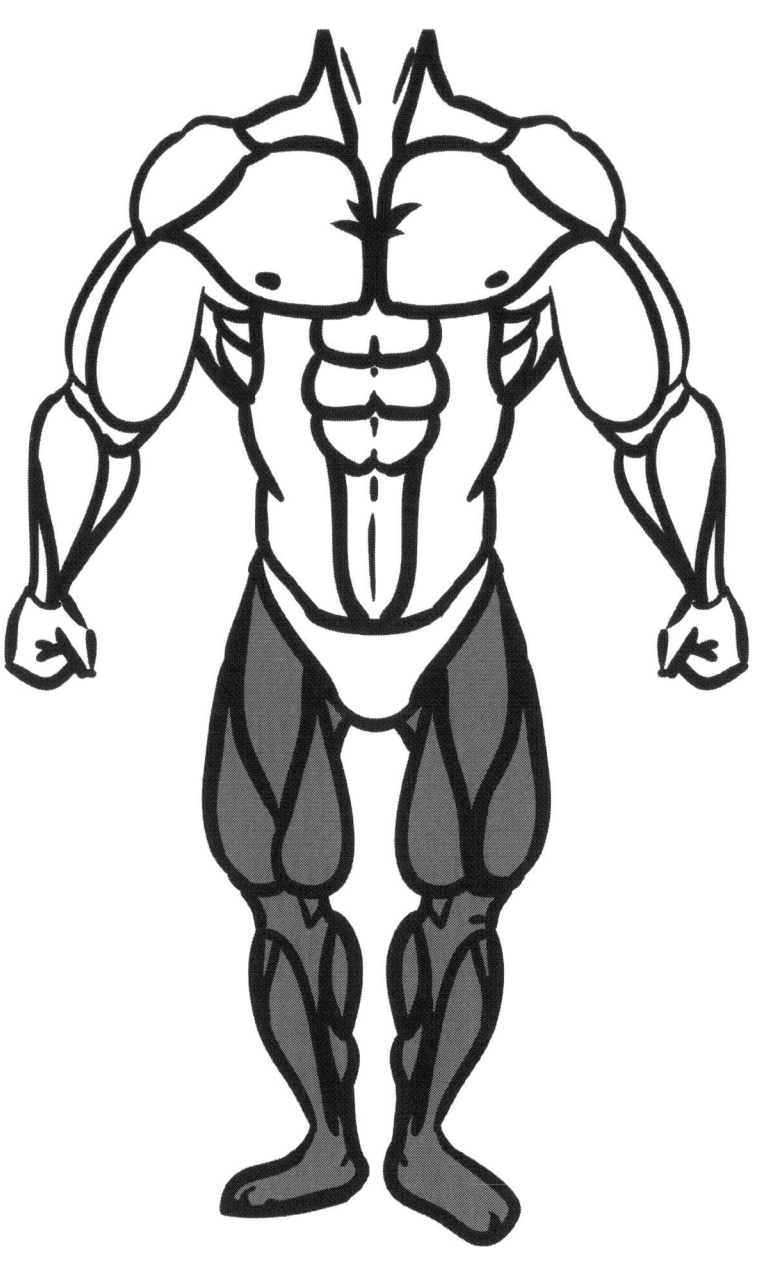

Open / Close Gates

This is a staple mobility exercise for elite athletes across a whole range of sports, so it is well worth adding into your routine.

Perform: 8-10 repetitions on each leg.

1. Stand upright and raise one leg upwards, knee bent at 90 degrees.

2. Bring the leg out to the side to open up your hips and groin.

3. Perform the same movement in reverse, first bringing the leg up to the side, then around to the front and back down to the ground.

Variation: You can also perform this exercise on your hands and knees, lifting one knee off the ground, extending it backwards and then bringing it all the way back round the front, and vice versa.

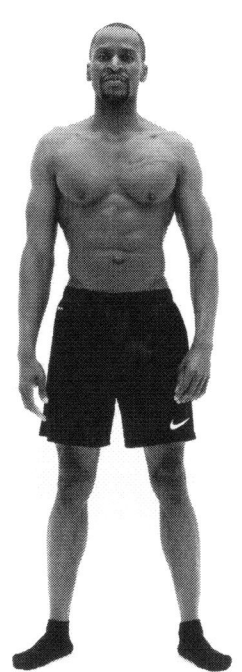 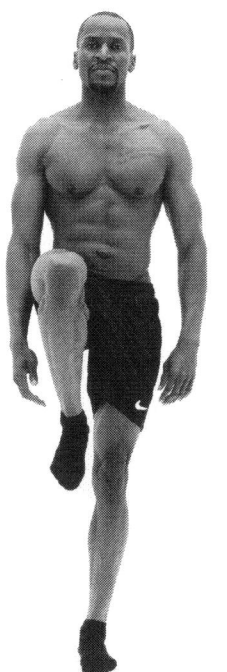 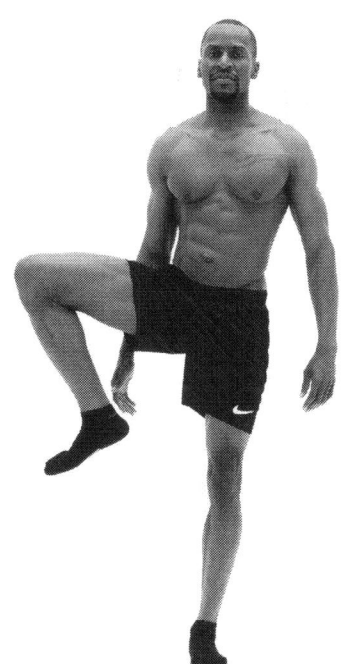

4. Warm-Up & Preparation   -   Mobility / Motion

Deep Squat

The squat is an exercise in itself, but we can make it – and almost every other lower body exercise – more effective by practicing the deep squat routinely. Because this one takes a little longer than the others you may prefer to do it on off days or after a heavy lower body session.

Perform: 3-5 minutes or more hold time.

1. Stand with your feet just beyond shoulder width apart, toes pointing out slightly at a comfortable, neutral angle.

2. Bend your knees and lower down into a squat position, ensuring you keep your lower back straight and push your hips back while doing so.

3. Once in position, clasp your hands together and rest your elbows just inside your knees, creating leverage to push your legs outward slightly.

4. Hold for 5 minutes, or as long as you can comfortably.

Variation: If you struggle to maintain your balance at first, place your legs either side of a sturdy pole or fixture and hold onto that to ensure you maintain the proper form.

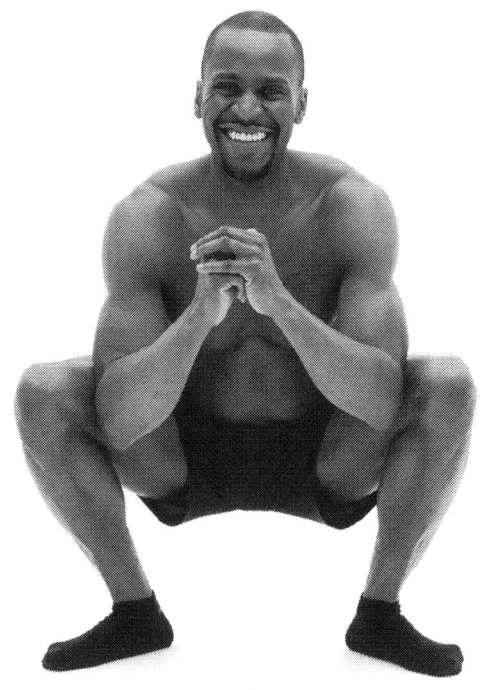

Lower Body

MOUNTAIN CLIMBERS

This is a fantastic, and dynamic, movement to warm up your body and get the blood flowing. Keep your reps unbroken and really lean into the movement to achieve the maximum benefit and increase your hip mobility.

Perform: 8 reps.

1. Assume the push-up position with your arms completely locked out, bringing your left leg forward and placing your foot beside your left hand.

2. Push both feet off the ground and quickly switch them. Now your right foot should be forward and your left out back. This counts as one rep.

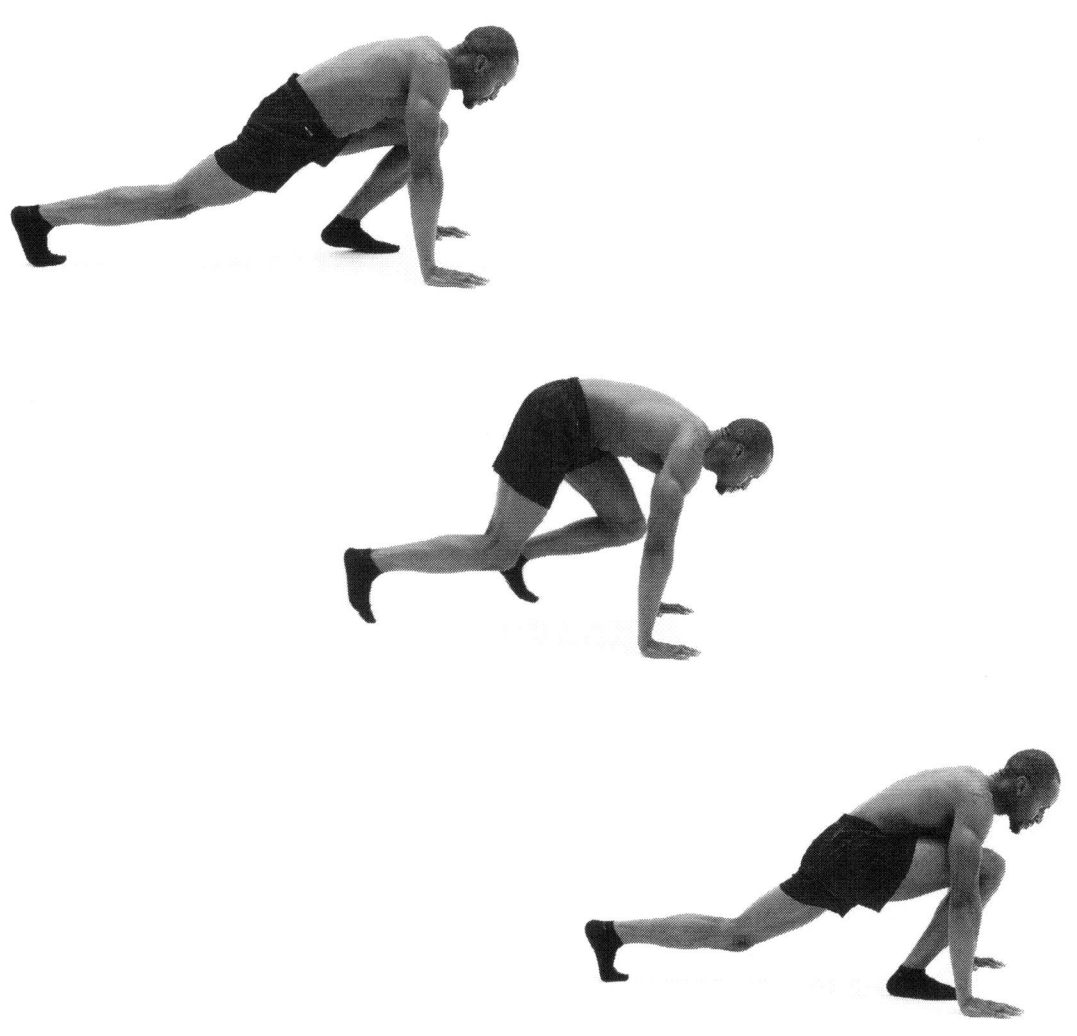

Frog Hops

This is another excellent exercise to improve your hip mobility, and prepare your body for any exercise involving the lower body.

Perform: 8 reps.

1. Assume the push-up position with arms fully locked out.

2. Leave your hands in place, and jump forward with your feet, landing with them just outside your hands.

3. Reverse the movement and return to the start to complete one rep.

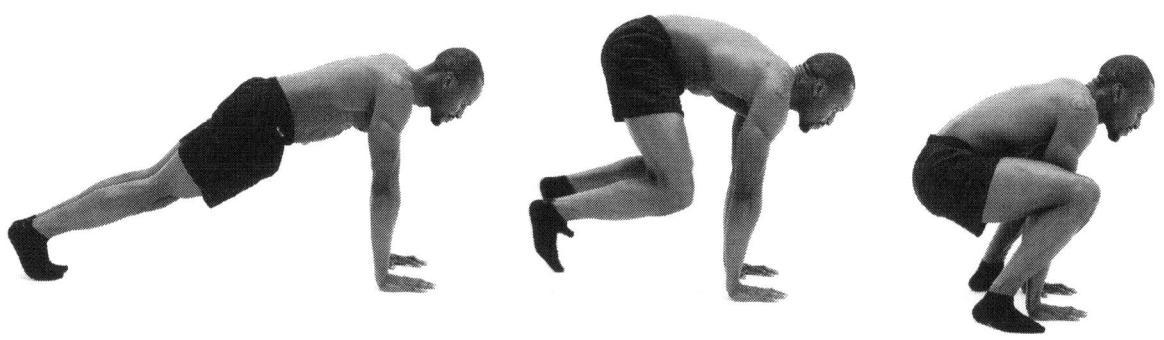

FLEXIBILITY & STRETCHING

Flexibility is a key component of a wide range of motion and, therefore, strength. Static stretching is the act of holding certain positions, generally for 15-30 seconds, in order to increase flexibility and minimize risk of injury.

You should be stretching after your workout or, if you are feeling tight in certain areas pre-workout, stretch them out then. Check out the following examples to target each area of your body. You can also do this on off days to accelerate your progress.

Remember: If you still feel tight in certain areas after stretching, throw in another set.

Tip: Relax during stretching. This might sound counter-productive but it is relaxing the muscles that allow them to stretch further. Try letting out a long, deep breath as you stretch a muscle and feel how much further it takes you!

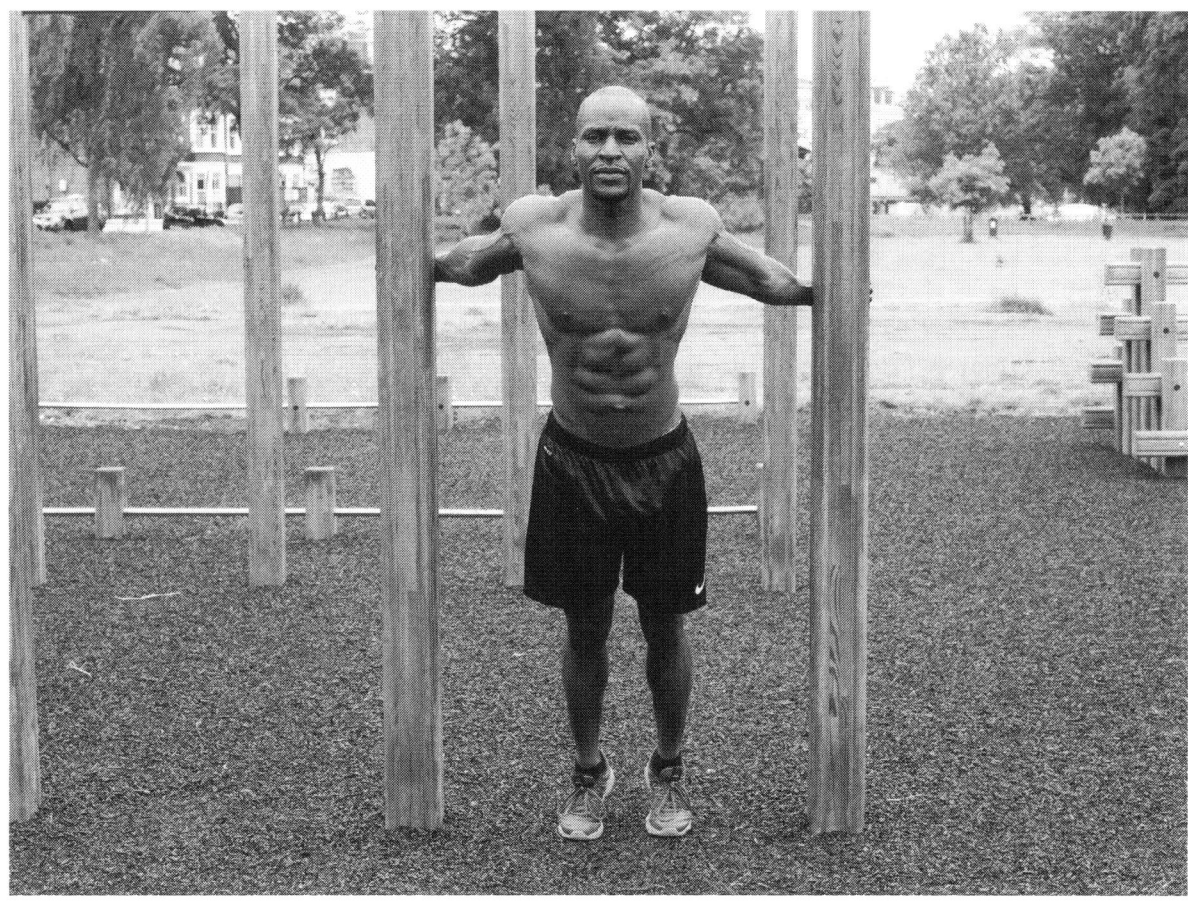

Upper Body

The upper body takes a beating during calisthenics training, so ensuring you are fully prepped is key. By improving your flexibility you will also get more out of your workouts, therefore enjoying greater results. We'll start from the top and work our way down.

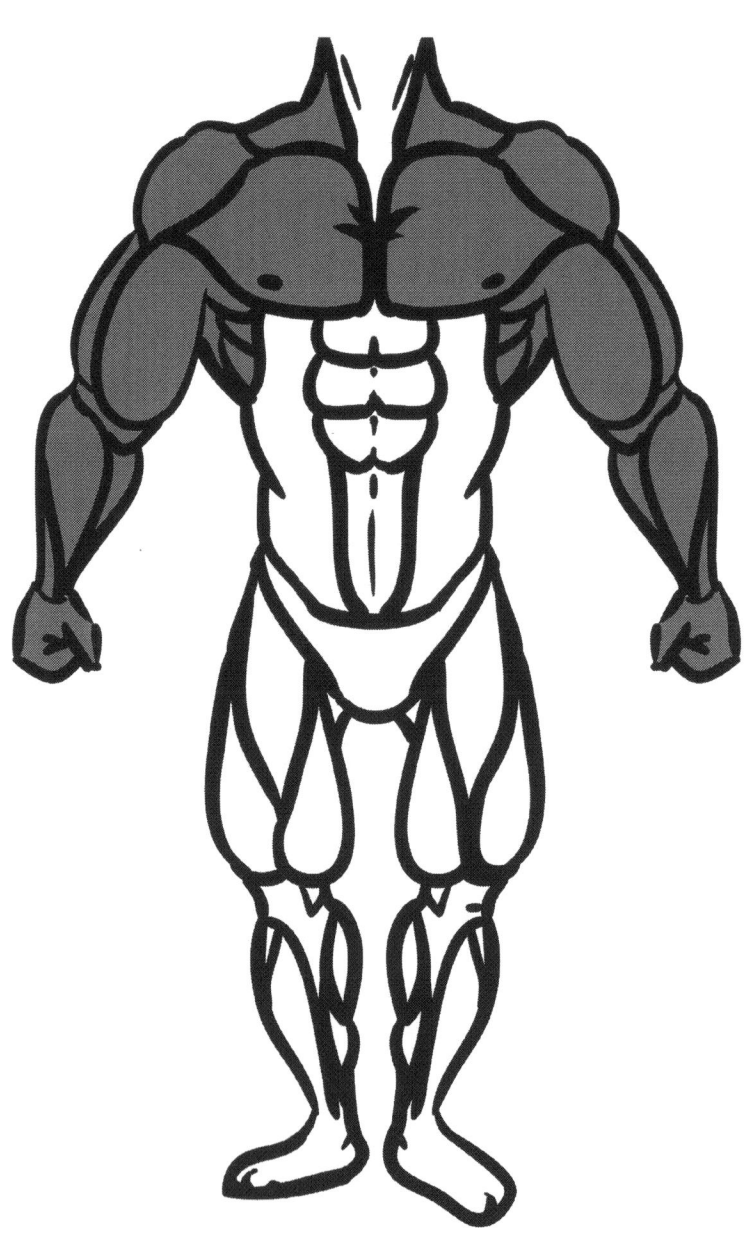

Upper Body

WRISTS & FOREARMS

Great as preparation for handstands as well as all-round strength, get to know both these variations to strengthen your wrists.

Perform: 30 second hold time.

1. Get on your knees and place your palms flat, fingers facing forward, just in front of your knees.

2. Lock your arms and slowly lean forwards as far as you can without raising your palms, and hold for the allotted time.

3. Return to start position and repeat the exercise, this time with your fingers facing towards you and leaning backwards instead of forwards.

Variation: If you find this too difficult then use a wall to perform a similar stretch.

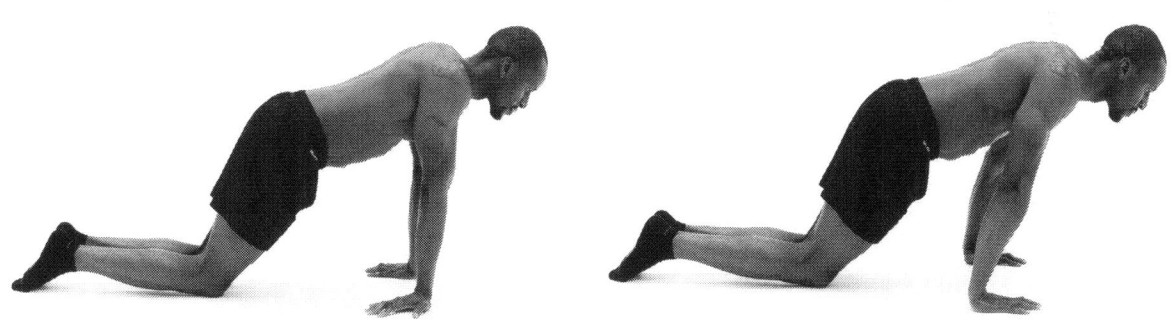

Chest & Shoulders

This stretch is essential in opening up two of the largest muscle groups in your upper body. Find somewhere comfortable and relax into it.

Perform: 30 second hold time.

1. Get onto your hands and knees, then stretch your arms out in front of you.

2. With your hands and knees rooted to the spot, bring your chest down towards the ground, exhaling as you go.

3. When your chest and shoulders are as low as possible, hold this pose for the allotted time. Remember to relax.

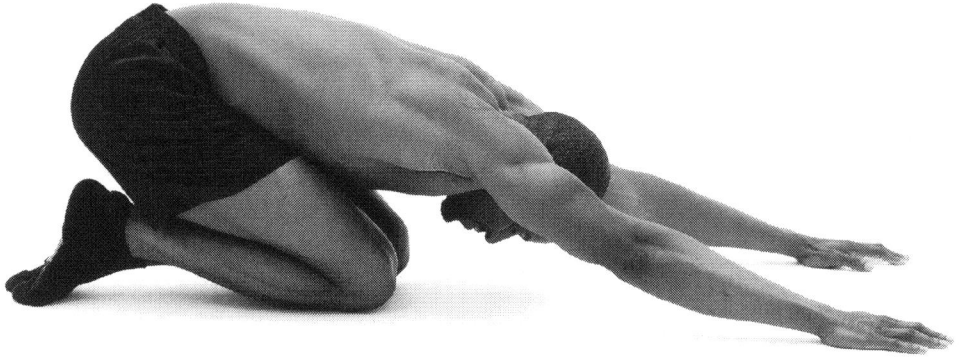

Upper Body

CHEST II

Your chest bears the brunt of almost every upper body exercise in calisthenics, so keep it properly conditioned with this simple stretch.

Perform: 30 second hold time.

You will need: upright parallel bars or doorframe.

1. Stand between the bars or doorframe and stretch your arms out to the sides, placing your palms flat on the surface.

2. Ensuring your arms stay straight, lean forward and stretch out your chest, holding for the allotted time.

Variations:

• If you don't have parallel bars use a single bar to stretch one side at a time. Instead of leaning forward, simply turn your body away from your affixed hand to stretch out one side of your chest then repeat on the other.

• You can also perform this exercise on a flat surface, rooting one hand against it and rotating away from that hand.

• Place a medicine ball or other platform on the floor and kneel beside it. Place one arm up on the platform, and then lower your body down to stretch out that side of your chest.

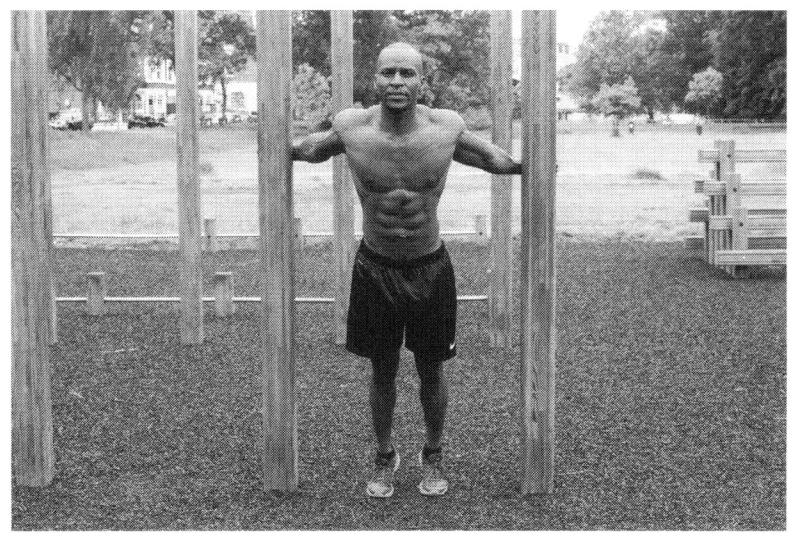

4. Warm-Up & Preparation   -   Flexibility & Stretching

UPPER BACK

This is another area that will take a beating as you condition your body, so get into the habit of stretching it out.

Perform: 30 second hold time.

You will need: a study bar or fixture.

1. Grab a straight bar or other immovable fixture with one hand.

2. Keeping your arm locked, slowly lean back to stretch out your lattisumus dorsi (lat) on that side.

3. Bring your free arm around in front of your body to stretch further and hold for the allotted time. Repeat on the other side for an effective back stretch.

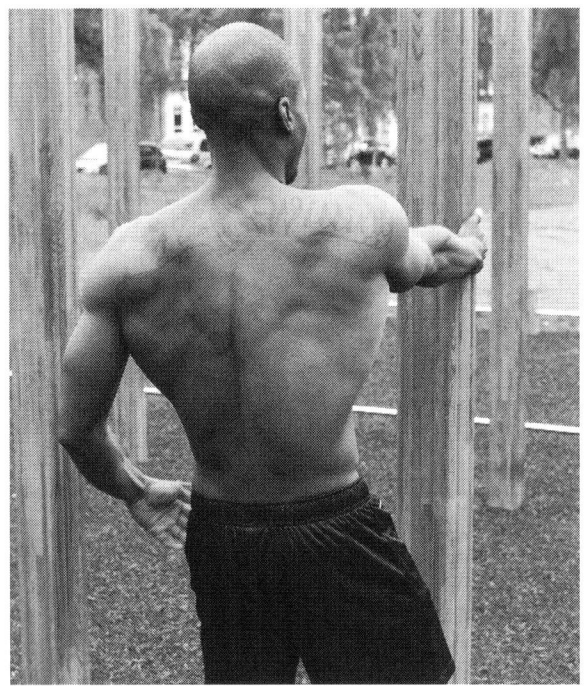
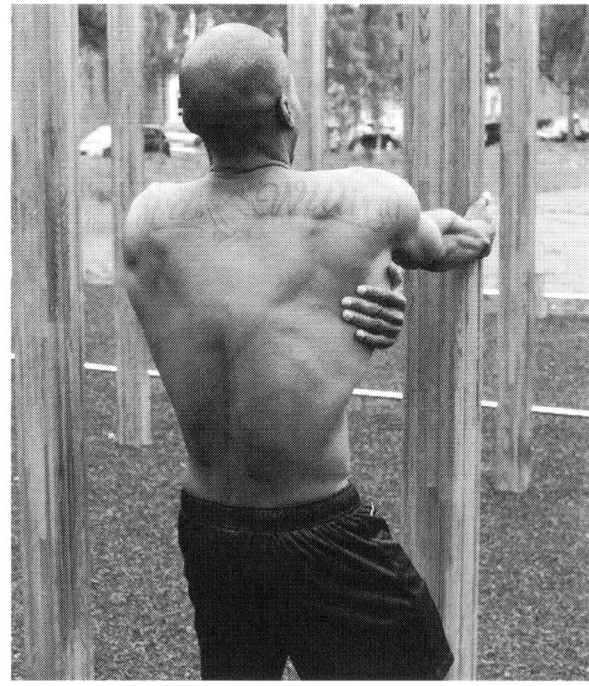

CORE

Everyone covets a chiseled core, and combining mobility and flexibility exercises with bodyweight training will help you achieve just that. You'll find this part quick and easy.

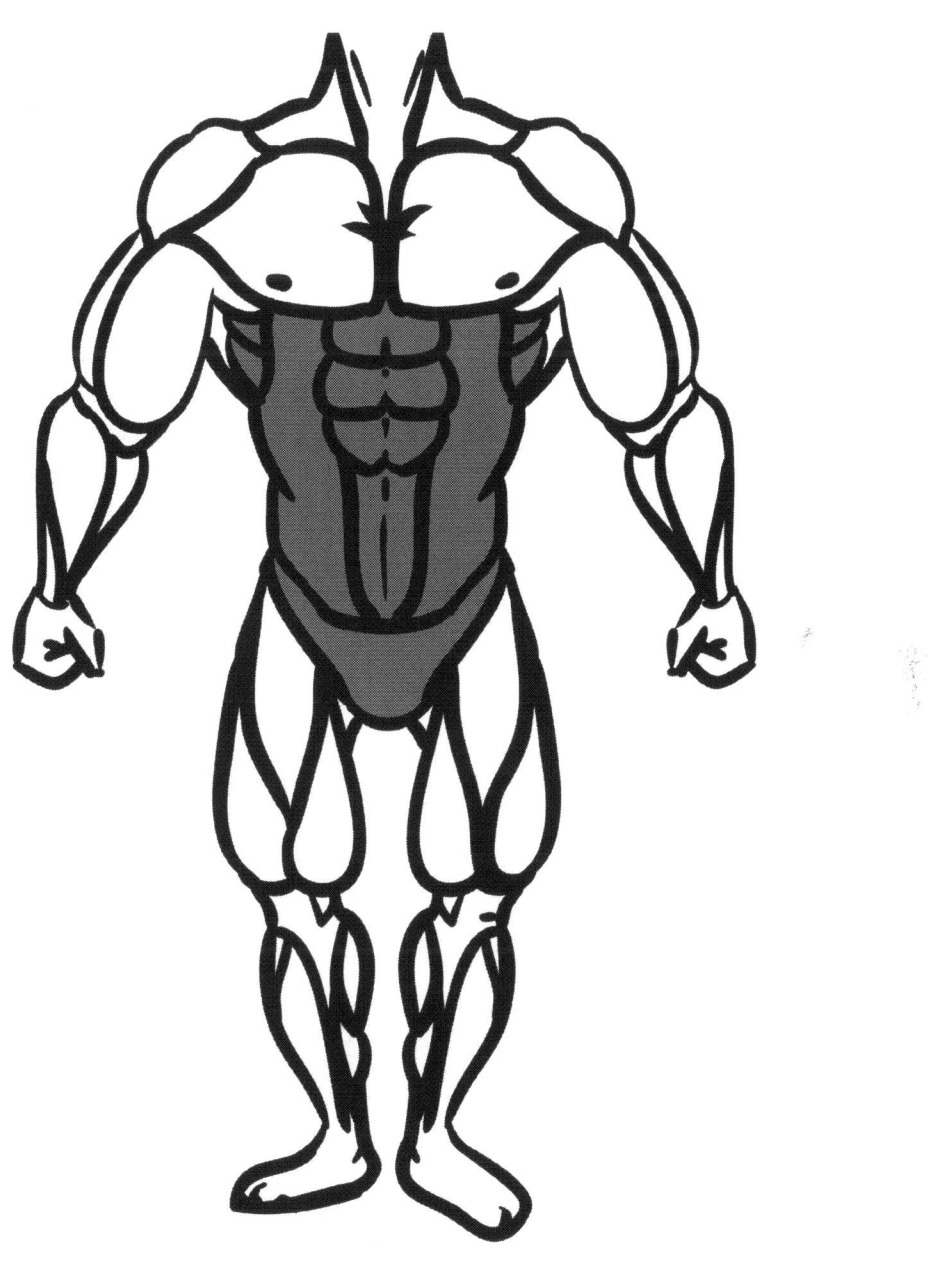

SIDE STRETCH

Prepare your lats, obliques, and lower back for movement with this standing side stretch, the same movement covered in mobility previously. As with all stretches, you don't want to be flexing, or straining against the movement. Instead, let your muscles relax and fall into the stretch for maximum benefit.

Perform: 15 second holds per side.

You will need: a long, lightweight bar.

1. Stand upright with your feet just wider than shoulder-width apart, grasping the bar over your head.

2. Keeping your arms straight, feet rooted and shoulders in position, lean over to one side to stretch out the other.

3. When you have reached as low as possible, reverse the movement and repeat the exercise on the other side of your body.

Variation: You can perform this exercise without a bar if needs be, simply lean over to one side and grab your leg with the closest hand, bringing the other arm up overhead.

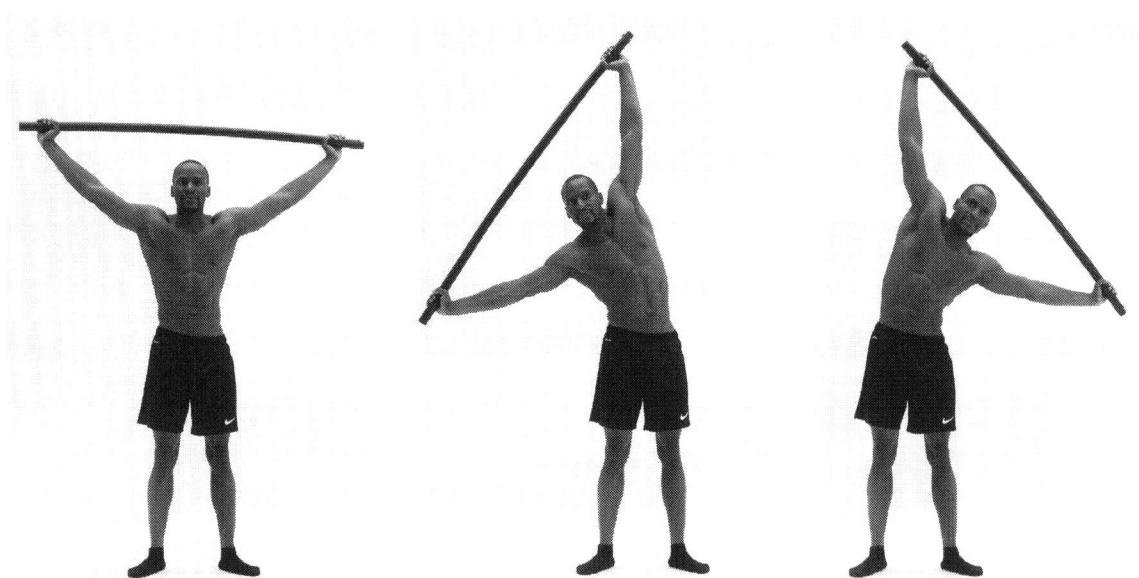

COBRA

If you've ever done yoga you'll know this one as the 'cobra' already. For everyone else, here it is, ideal for opening up your lower back and hips.

Perform: 15-30 second hold time.

1. Lie on your stomach and place your palms flat on the floor, similar to a standard push-up position, fingers facing forward, about shoulder-width apart.

2. With your hips rooted to the ground, raise your head and look upwards, allowing your spine to arch and hold for allotted time.

Variation: If you find this tough to hold, practice raising up onto your forearms and holding the stretch there first.

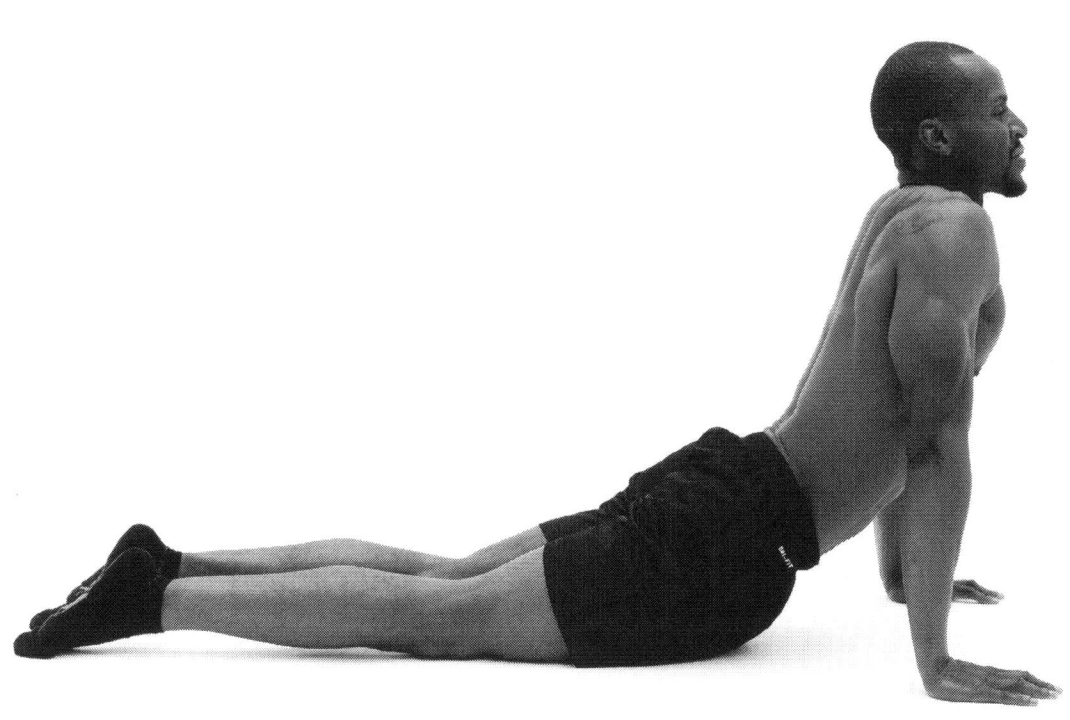

Cat

Another yoga stretch named 'cat', essentially designed to stretch the opposite way to cobra, opening up your back nicely.

Perform: 15-30 second hold time.

1. Get on your hands and knees, palms flat directly underneath your shoulders, fingers facing forward.

2. Drop your head and arch your back as if trying to look at your naval, and hold for the allotted amount of time.

Variation: To turn this into a mobility exercises, get into position and then transition to a downwardly arched back, raising your head up. Moving between the two in a fluid motion is a great way to warm up.

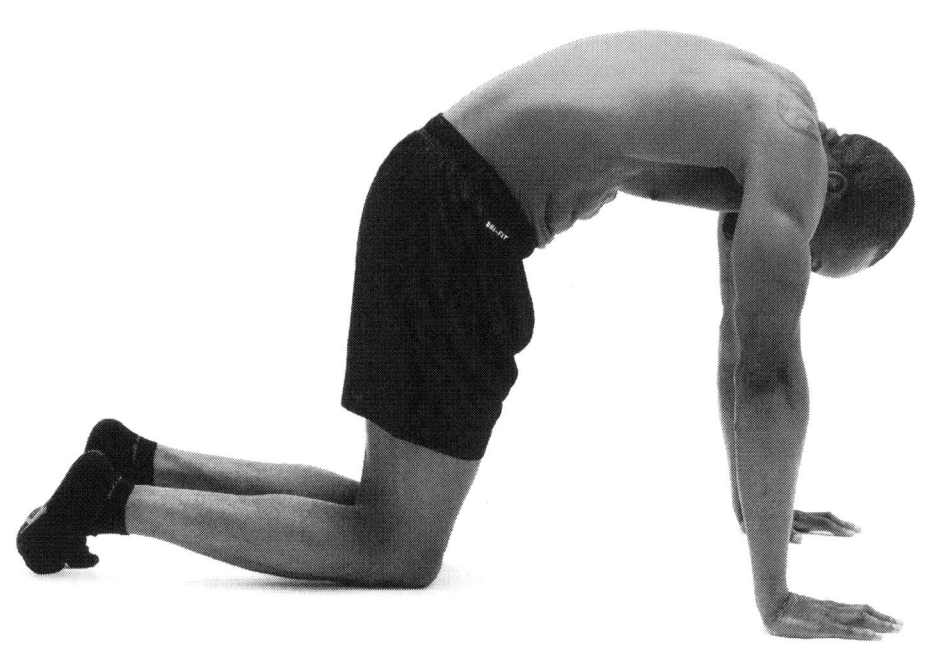

LOWER BODY

Last but by no means least is lower body flexibility. Not only will this help you achieve your dream body, it will also prove useful in everyday life, especially as the years go by. Don't let tight hamstrings, hip flexors or other problem areas hold you back. Let's go!

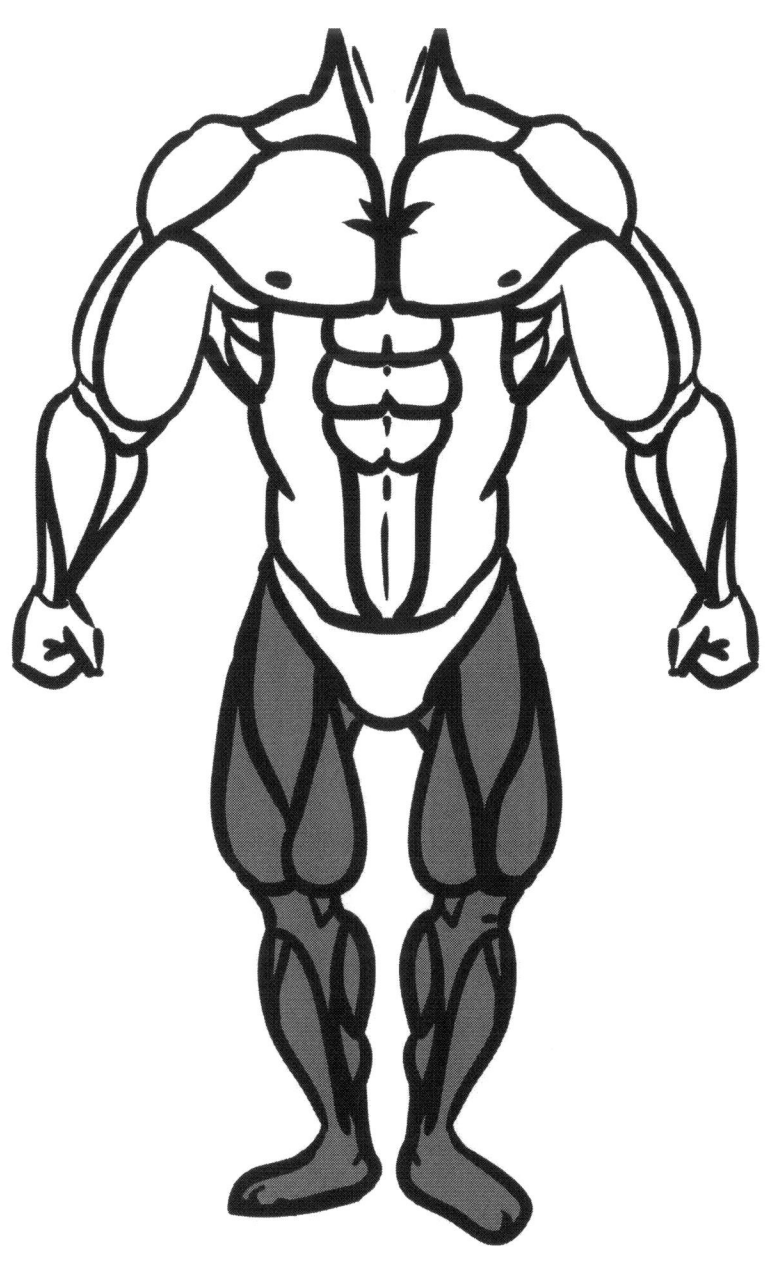

4. Warm-Up & Preparation - Flexibility & Stretching

CALVES

Essential for strength and stability, you must ensure your calves are flexible enough to cope with the demands of calisthenics. And, of course, for showing off at barbeques!

Perform: 30 seconds hold time for each leg.

1. Get into push-up position.

2. Take one foot and rest the top of it on the heel of the other.

3. Slowly push the heel of the standing foot down as far as possible and hold for allotted time.

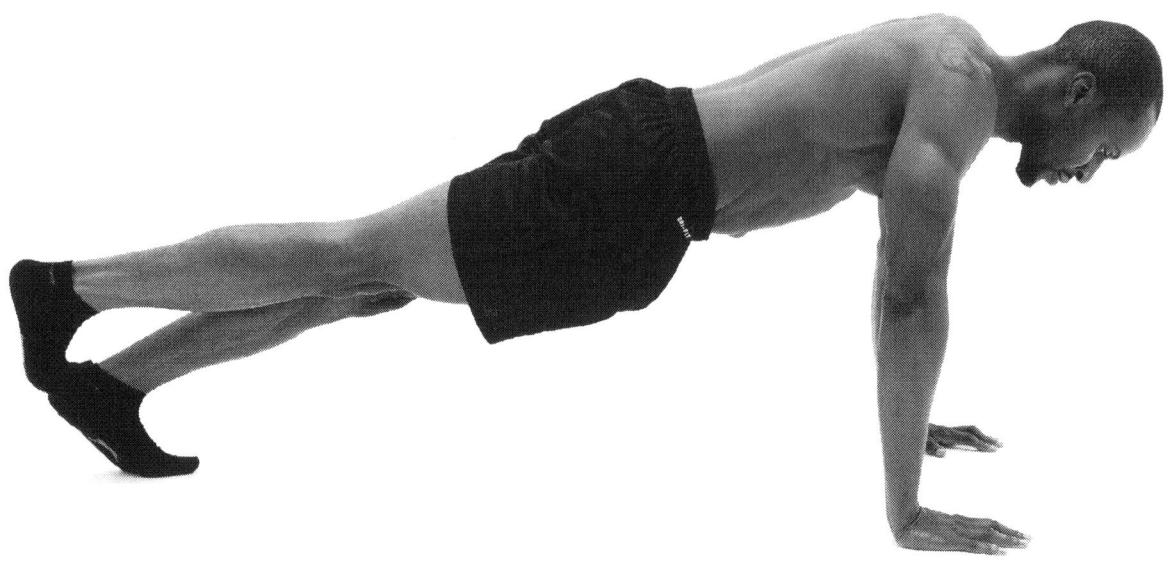

Lower Body

HAMSTRINGS

Most people have tight hamstrings, which can severely inhibit your range of lower body motion. Loosen them up like so:

Perform: 30 second hold time on each leg.

1. Sit down with both legs stretched out in front of you, toes pointing upwards.

2. Bring one foot towards you so the sole is against the inner thigh of the other leg.

3. Keeping your back straight, lean forwards towards the toes of your outstretched leg and hold for allotted time.

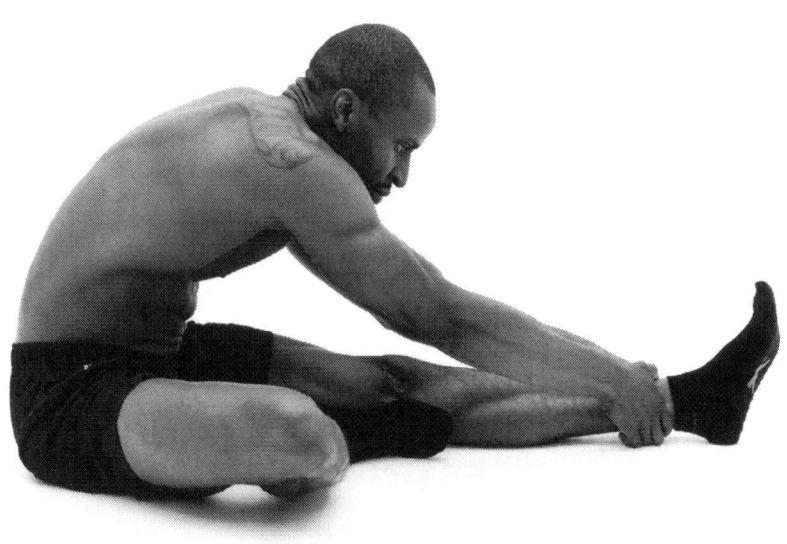

GROIN

Opening up your groin will also open up your hips. You are probably beginning to see how everything is linked together now, so you should never neglect one area in favor of another.

Perform: 30 second hold time.

1. Sit down and bring the soles of your feet together.

2. Keeping your back straight, pull your feet towards your body as close as possible.

3. Try to move your knees outwards to touch the floor. If you cannot do this with leg power alone, use your elbows or hands for a little assistance.

4. Hold for allotted time. You may find one side tighter than the other here, but don't worry, it will even out over time.

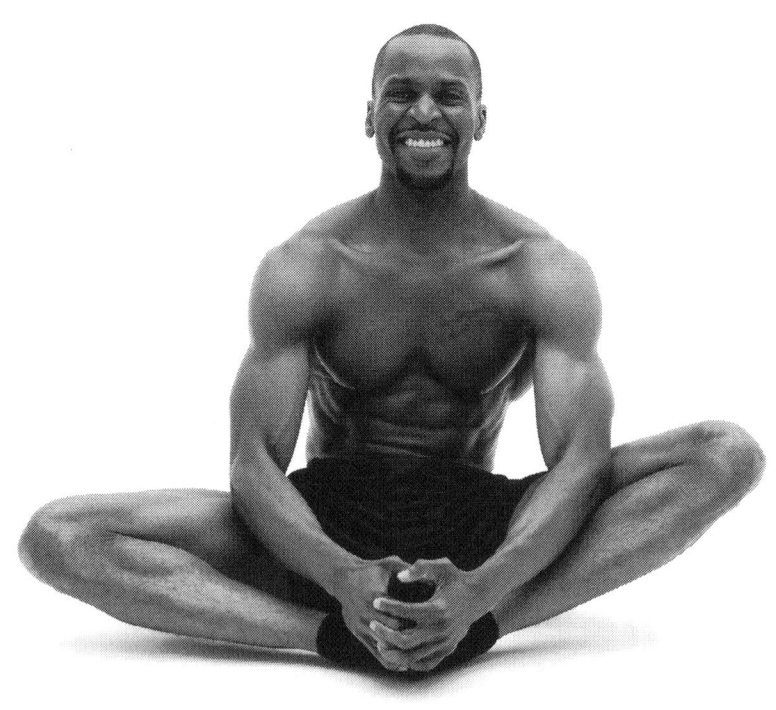

Lower Body

GLUTES

This is a hugely powerful part of your body, driving some of the most important motions required for lower body activities, which is why professional athletes and sports stars often have backsides like Beyoncé.

Perform: 30 second hold time on each side.

1. Lay on your back.

2. Bend the knee of one leg and bring it towards you, grasping the leg underneath your hamstring area with both hands.

3. Bring the other leg up and over so the ankle is resting just above the knee of the leg you are holding.

4. Pull the leg you are holding towards you to create a stretch in the opposite side and hold for allotted time.

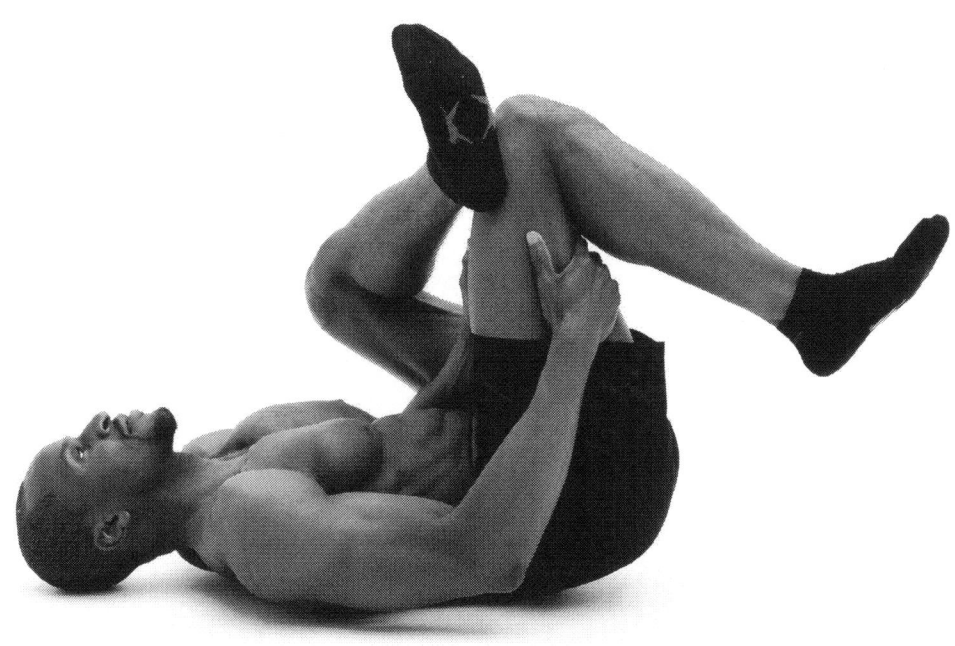

Hip Flexor

Your hip flexors work in harmony with your glutes so you can't stretch one without the other. Check this out:

Perform: 30 second hold time on each side

1. Stand upright, then place one foot forward.

2. Bend the knee of your front foot and, keeping your body straight and rear foot on the spot, lean forward.

3. When you feel a stretch in the top of your back leg, hold for allotted time.

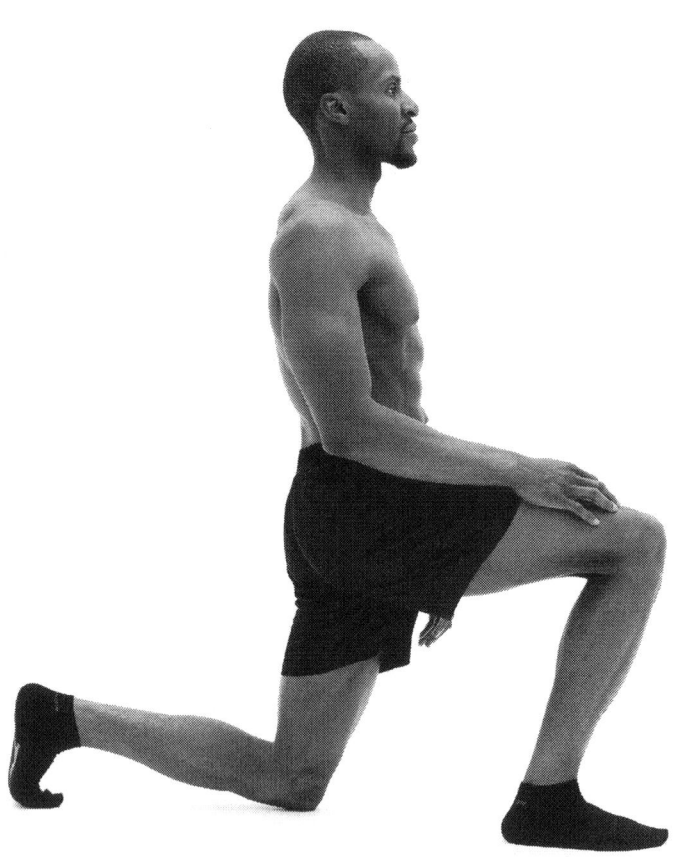

Hips II

Here, we'll focus on your hips, groin, and hammies, areas that are chronically tight in many people.

Perform: 30 second hold.

1. Start at a comfortable sitting position on the floor, and then spread your legs outward as far as you can.

2. Slowly lean forward as far as possible into the space between your legs, and hold for allotted time.

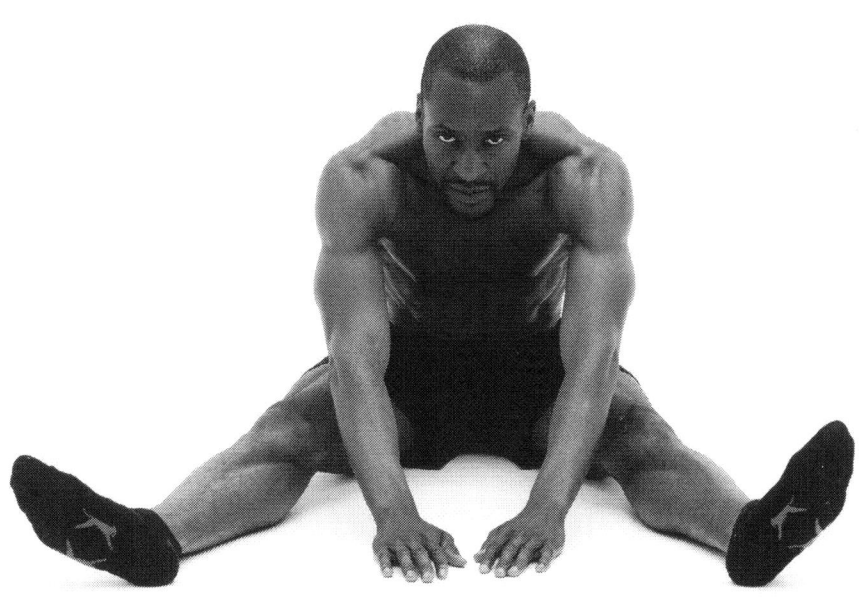

QUADRICEPS

Another massive muscle group vitally important to both calisthenics and day-to-day life are your quads. Keep them happy with this simple stretch:

Perform: 30 second hold time.

1. Lie down flat on your stomach.

2. Bend one knee and bring the foot towards your glutes.

3. Grasp the foot with your hand and pull it towards your glutes, then hold for allotted time.

That covers the essential stretching for major muscle groups. Remember to stretch after each workout to aid recovery and increase range of motion and, subsequently, strength.

Listen to your body and seek advice from a specialist if you are unsure about anything. You should be using this advice as a general guideline to help build your own stretching routine rather than sticking to it exactly as it's written above.

For a comprehensive guide on building superhuman strength through flexibility, pick up our companion book on Amazon. Just search 'Pure Calisthenics Flexibility'.

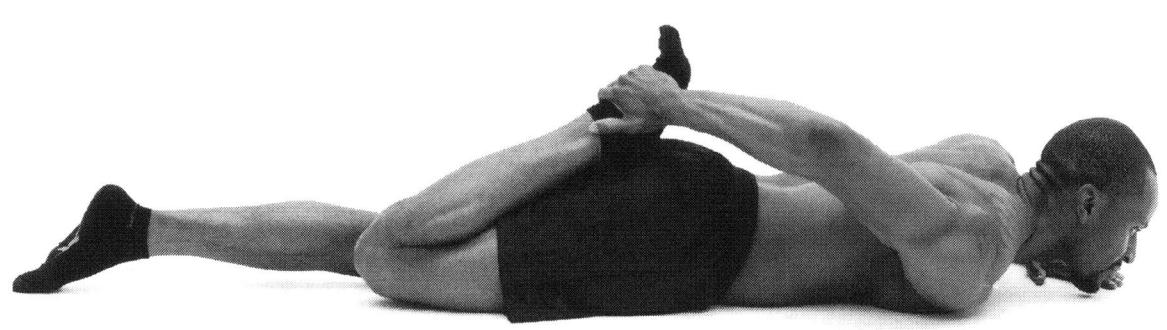

"Take care of your body. It's the only place you have to live."

Jim Rohn

5. Exercises

It's time to get into the good stuff! If you commit to mastering the following exercises and don't throw in the towel when the going gets tough then you WILL experience mind-blowing results.

Disclaimer: This bodyweight training guide has been designed to help you learn the art of calisthenics progressively. Each exercise will start off with the simplest variation, becoming more difficult as you work through the book.

Since we cannot be there to train you in person, we have provided HD photographs and detailed tutorials. We cannot be held accountable for any misuse of instructions or injuries that occur as a result. It is down to you to be smart and attempt only what you are ready for.

Where possible, always use a spotter or personal trainer to ensure you are using the correct form for each exercise. There is no glory or value in squeezing out more sets or reps than someone else if you aren't performing the exercises properly.

Remember: This is a resource created to teach bodyweight exercises, NOT a training program. We cannot suggest an exact amount of sets and reps for you without knowing your level of ability, so the numbers given in this guide are just a suggestion.

If you want to get started with a proper training routine you will find a link at the back of this book to our free companion program. As always, for a more personal approach, hook up with a calisthenics trainer to create a bespoke program.

All that is left to do at this stage is make sure you are sufficiently warmed up before jumping into any of the following exercises. If you skipped the section on warm-up and preparation, do yourself a favor and go back a few steps. It might just be the difference between make or break.

So, you're clued up, you're warmed up, and you're raring to go. Just what kind of crazy exercises are we going to use to achieve SUPERHUMAN form?

Well, the most astonishing thing is, it all starts with the humble sit-up.

Let's do this!

CORE

When it comes to calisthenics your core really is the star of the show. It may look like your upper and lower body are bearing the brunt of it, but everything is linked in the center so it is absolutely essential to pay special attention to developing core strength.

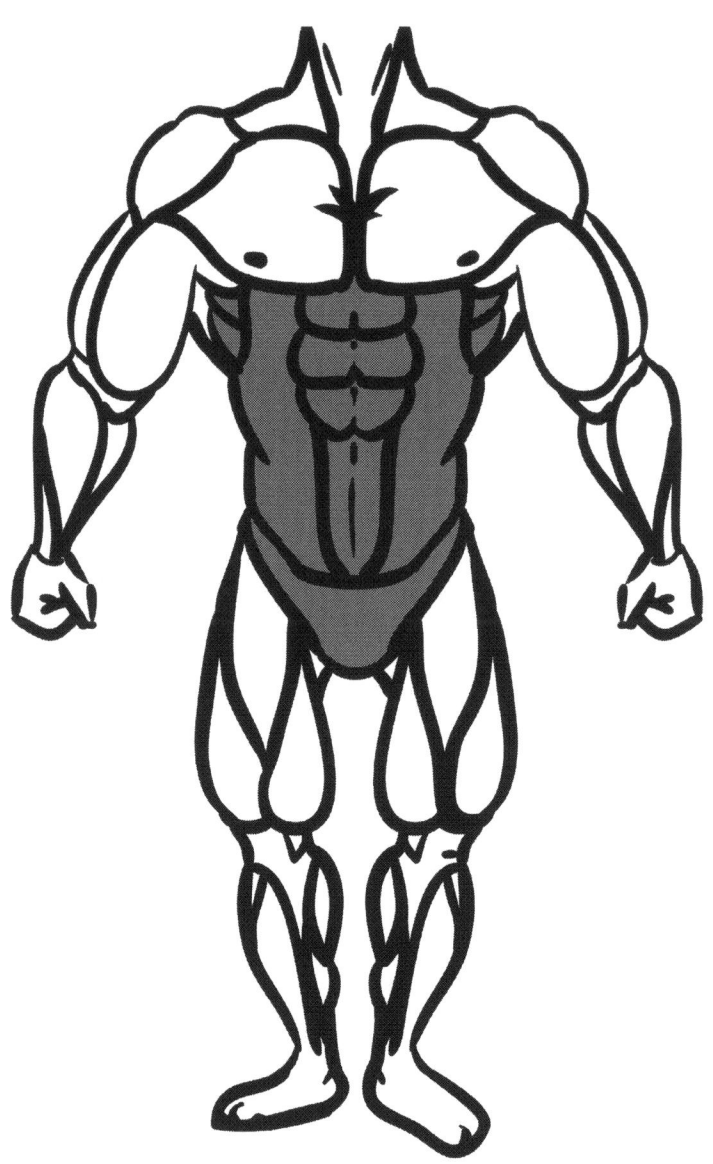

Fundamentals

Don't ignore the core! As the name suggests, your core is at the hub of all exercises, and you must keep it finely tuned if you want to build the perfect body. Progress through these fundamentals to achieve a popping six-pack and shredded stomach in quick time!

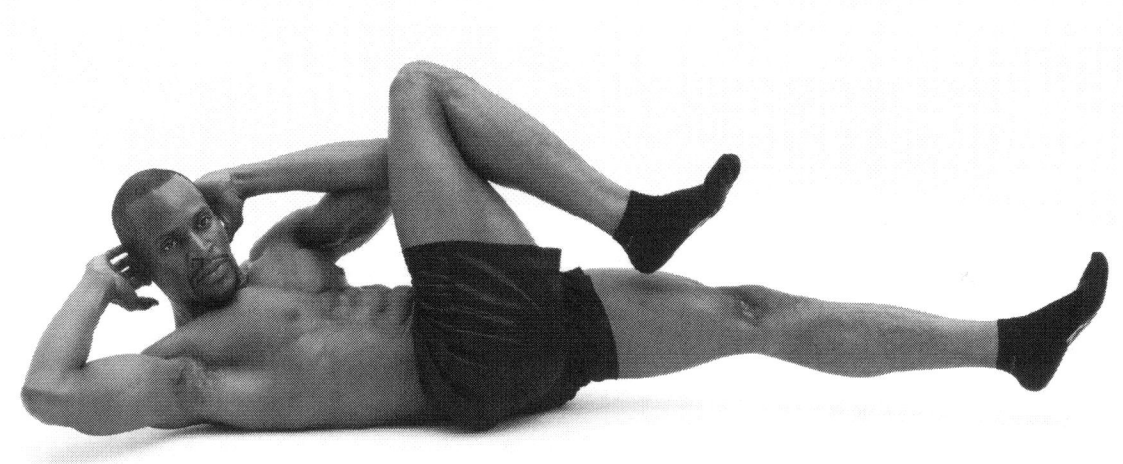

SIT-UP

This classic core exercise has been the foundation of training programs for as long as they have existed, so it's well worth mastering early on.

NB: Proper form is essential with all exercises, but it is especially important where the core is concerned, since you will also be calling your spine into action.

To maximize your results and avoid injury, always do as much as you can with the correct form instead of cheating to knock out another rep or two.

Perform: 3-4 sets of 10-20 reps.

1. Lie flat on your back with your knees bent at 90 degrees and feet flat on the floor. Place your toes under a secure surface if just starting out.

2. Place your fingertips against your temples and allow your arms to come parallel to the ground.

3. Contract your core and sit up as far as possible, aiming to bring your elbows past your knees.

4. When you have reached forward as far as possible, reverse the movement to complete one rep.

Variation: Have a buddy press your feet into the ground, or tuck them under something sturdy in order to generate greater leverage when you are just starting out.

Fundamentals

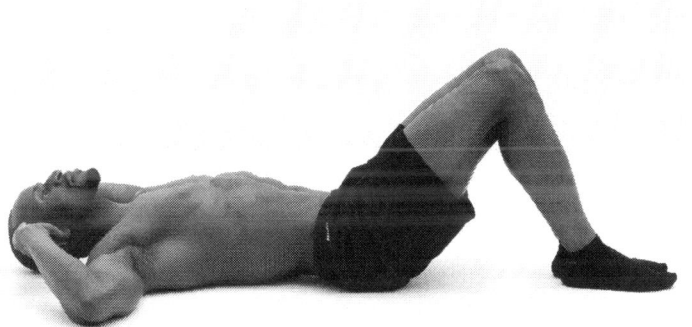

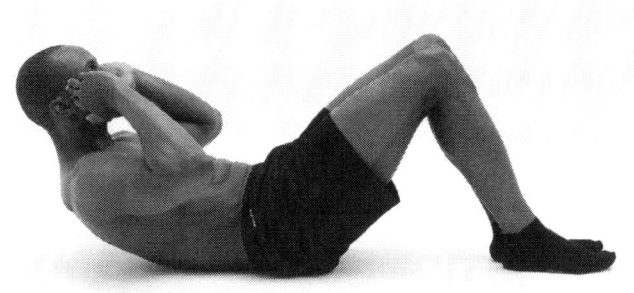

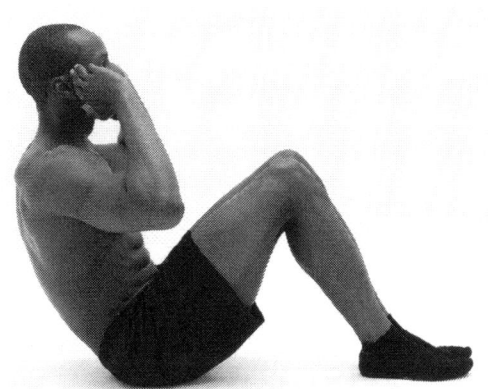

5. Exercises - Core

CRUNCH

The crunch is a fairly simple yet very effective way of strengthening your core and can be performed by beginners and experts alike.

Perform: 3-4 sets of 10-20 reps.

1. Lie on your back with your knees bent at approximately 90 degrees and your feet placed flat on the floor.

2. Place your hands loosely at the sides your head and, keeping your lower back and feet rooted to the ground, curl your shoulders and upper back forward towards your knees. The aim here is not to move far, but to feel a very concentrated 'crunch' within a small range of movement.

3. Lower your shoulders and upper back towards the ground again to complete one rep.

If you struggle to keep your feet flat on the ground during this exercise then place them under something secure until you are able to do the exercise properly.

Super important: do not use your hands to pull yourself up, as this will strain your neck. Instead, keep your chin tucked, hands loose and concentrate all the effort in your core.

If your neck is getting tired, it's because you are straining it to compensate for a weak core. Instead of yanking on your head, just perform fewer reps with the proper form.

Over time you will develop the core strength required to perform the allocated sets and reps, and you will find that your neck no longer seems to be a source of pain!

Fundamentals

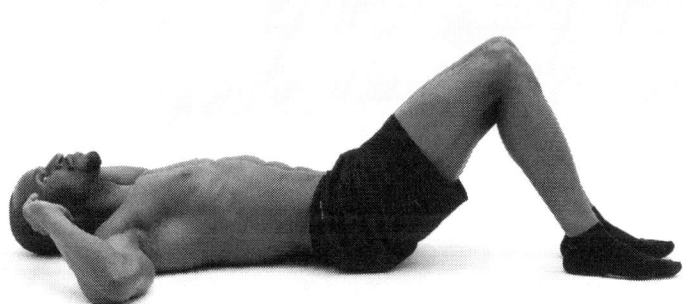

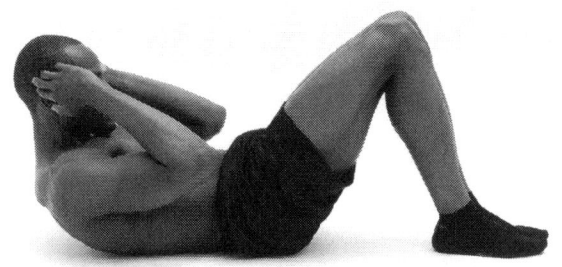

5. Exercises - Core

PLANK

The plank is a great core strength and stability exercise, and the chances are that you have already performed it before in some form or another.

Perform: 3-4 sets of 20-30 second hold times.

1. Get into regular push up position, but instead of placing your hands on the floor place your forearms flat against the floor straight out in front of you.

2. Balancing on your forearms and toes, raise your core until your body forms a straight line from your feet right through your knees, hips, and shoulders.

3. Hold this position for the allotted time or as long as possible to complete one set.

If you notice your back arching or your stomach sagging towards the ground, do your best to squeeze your abdominal muscles hard and keep your body in a straight line.

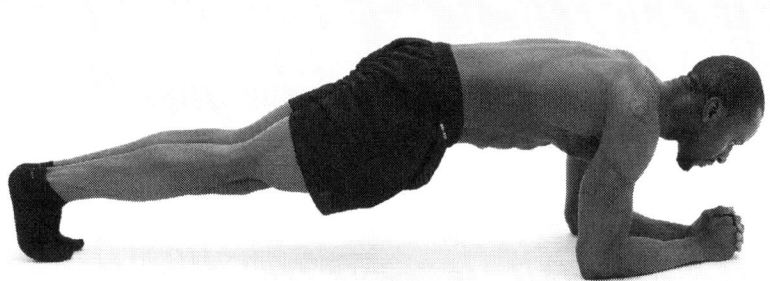

Fundamentals

SIDE PLANK

This exercise will do for your obliques what regular the regular plank does for your abs, and is another great foundation exercise for your core.

Perform: 3-4 sets of 20-30 second hold times per side.

1. Lie on your side and support your upper bodyweight with one forearm placed on the ground at a 90-degree angle relative to the rest of your body.

2. With your bottom foot on its side, bring the other foot to rest on top of it.

3. Bring your hips up off the ground so your body forms a straight line.

4. Hold this position for allotted time or as long as possible to complete one set.

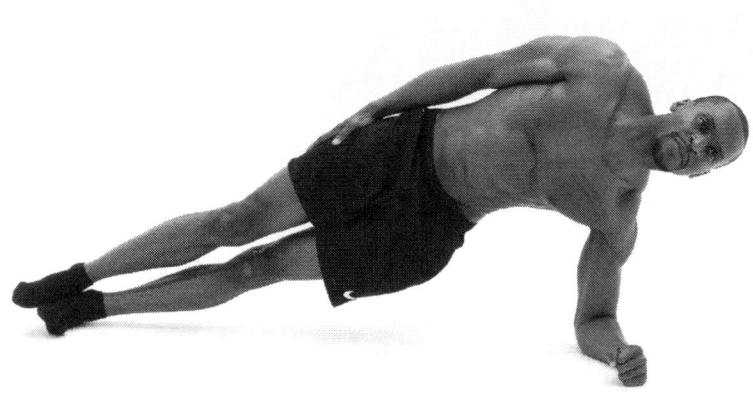

5. Exercises - Core

EXTENDED PLANK

The extended plank takes the standard plank position one step further, extending the arms further forward to provide a greater challenge.

Perform: 3-4 sets of 15-20 second hold times.

1. Assume the standard plank position.

2. Now move your hands forward until your chest is only a few inches from touching the ground. Keep your lower back straight.

3. Hold for a long as possible.

NB: There is no limit to the distance you can set out between your feet and hands here. Just go as far as you can without sacrificing form or touching the ground!

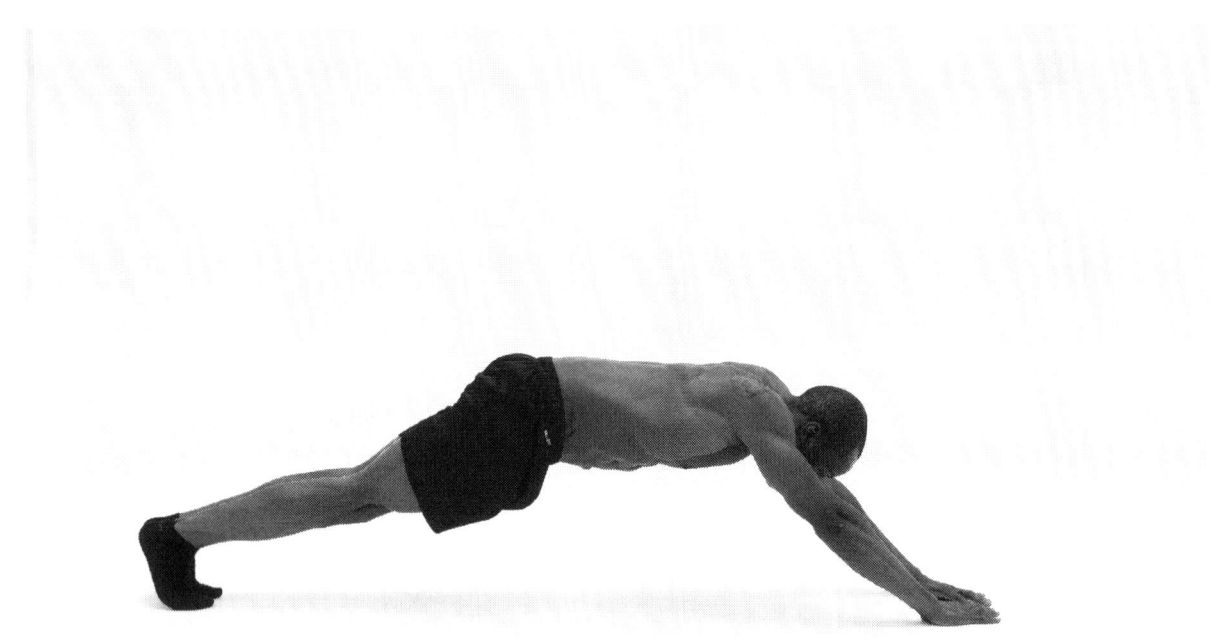

Bicycle Kicks

This gentle, dynamic movement is a fine way to strengthen your core and it also doubles as a brilliant warm-up for core and lower body sessions.

Perform: 3-4 sets of 20-30 seconds.

1. Lie flat on your back.

2. Bring one knee up towards your chest while extending the other out.

3. Switch legs in a continuous 'cycling' motion for the allotted time.

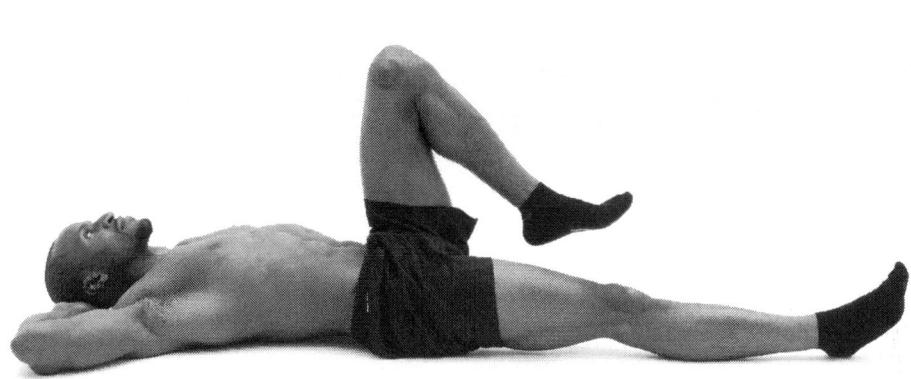

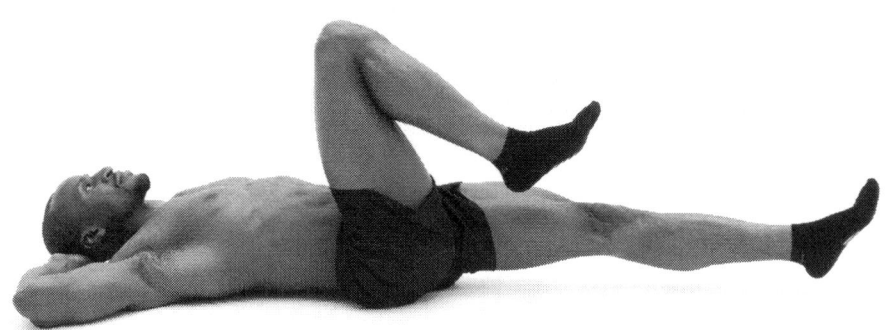

5. Exercises - Core

ELBOW TO KNEE CROSS

Think of this as a souped-up version of bicycle kicks. This will crunch your core in every direction and build popping abs and obliques!

Perform: 3-4 sets of 15-20 seconds.

1. Lay flat on your back, hands behind your head.

2. Bring one knee up and across your body.

3. Bring the opposite elbow around towards the knee.

4. Repeatedly switch elbows and knees for the allotted time. Feel the burn!

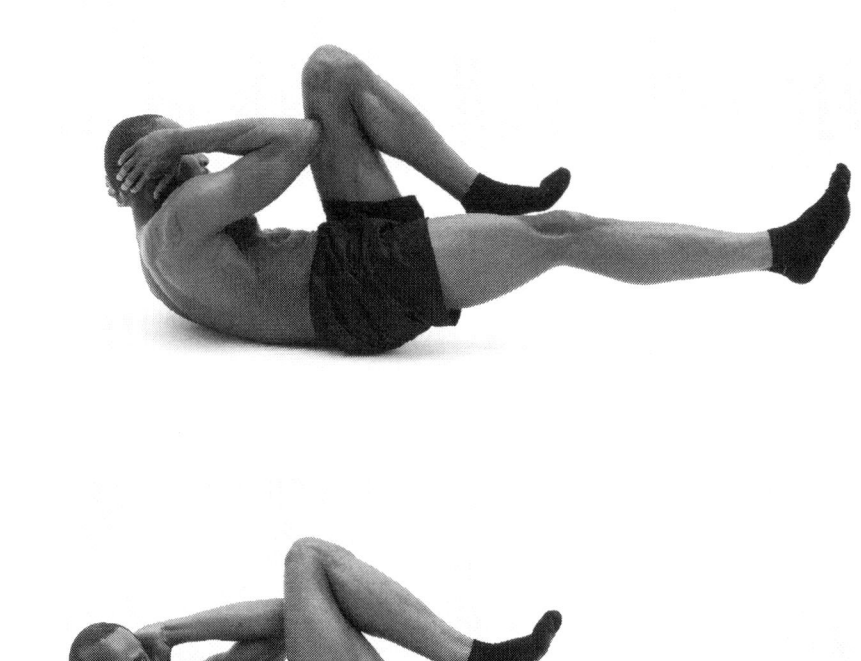

Russian Twists

This one is just as menacing as it sounds. Prepare to give your core a complete workout.

Perform: 3-4 sets of 20-30 seconds.

1. Sit on the floor with your legs bent at around a 90-degree angle and lean back a little.

2. Pivoting around your core and keeping a straight back, reach around and touch the floor on one side.

3. Repeat on the other side to complete a rep and continue without stopping until you hit your target or cannot do any more with the proper form.

Variations:

• Extend your feet further forward or lift them off the ground entirely for a greater challenge. If this badly affects your form, you may need to build up more core strength using the standard version first.

• Hold a weighted ball in your hands to up the intensity.

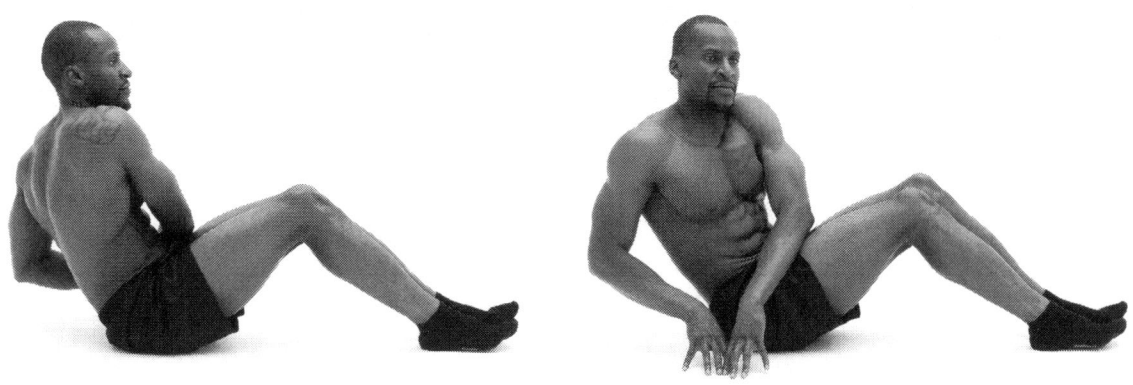

5. Exercises - Core

DISH HOLD

As you begin to develop your core for the more strenuous calisthenics exercise, the dish is an excellent addition to your routine.

No equipment required and easy to perform wherever you are, this is a favorite among calisthenics pros.

Perform: 3-4 sets of 15-20 second hold times.

1. Lie flat on the floor with your arms over your head

2. Raise your head, arms, and shoulders off the ground, and press into the ground with your lower back.

3. Raise your feet about a foot off the floor while keeping your legs straight.

4. Hold for the required time, and increase as it becomes easier with practice.

Remember, if you cannot manage the allotted time, split it into as many sets as it takes to hit the target, e.g. 2 x 10 secs = 20 secs.

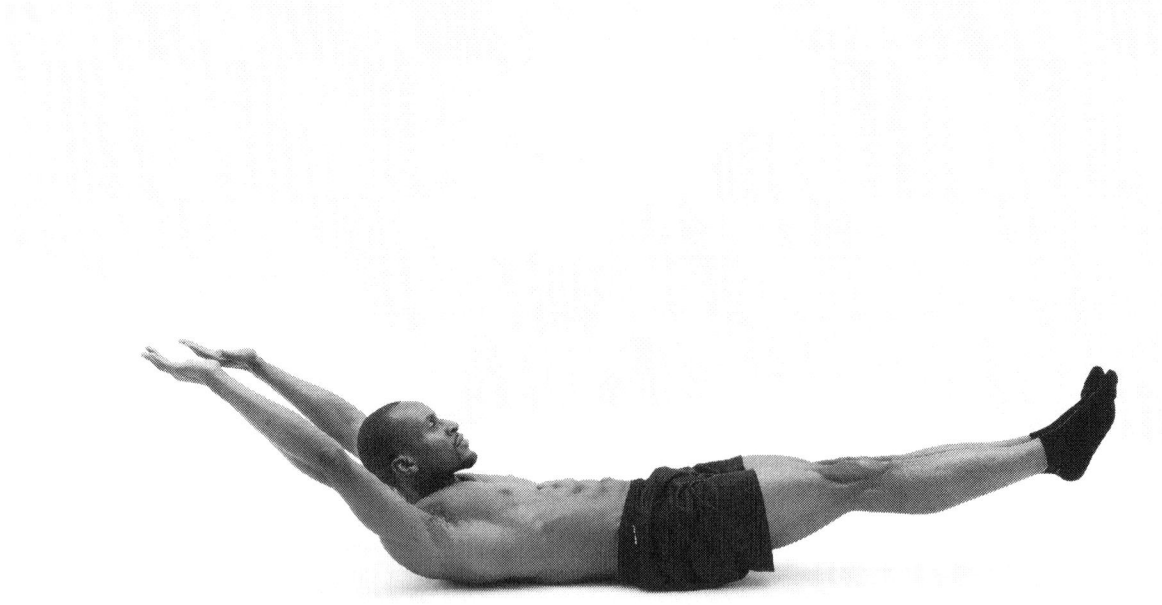

Fundamentals

V-Up

Once you're comfortable with the dish, you can bring motion into the equation with v-ups. Be sure to focus the tension in your core instead of straining your neck.

Perform: 3-4 sets of 10-15 reps.

1. Lie on your back with your arms by your sides and legs stretched out straight in front of you, feet slightly raised.

2. Lift your upper body off the ground while simultaneously bending your knees and bringing them up towards your chest. Keeping your arms and spine straight, aiming to move your hands past your knees.

3. When you have reached as far as possible, reverse the movement to complete one rep and go straight into the next.

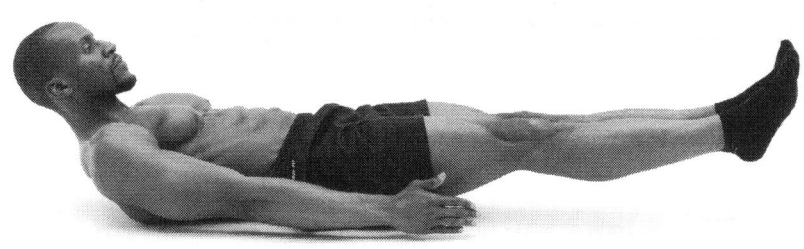

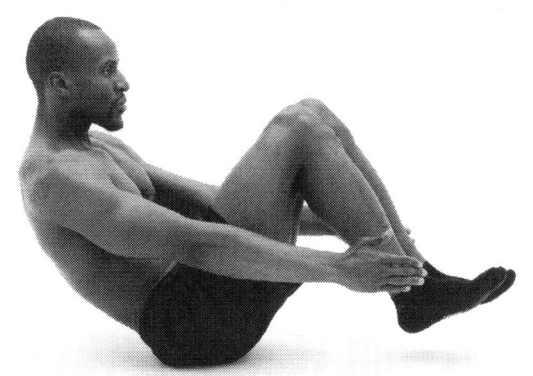

5. Exercises - Core

LYING LEG RAISES

This movement will target those hard to reach lower abdominal muscles, essential for core strength and good posture.

Perform: 3-4 sets of 15-20 reps.

1. Lie flat on your back with your legs stretched out in front of you, arms by your sides.

2. Keeping your upper body and lower back rooted to the floor and your legs straight, raise your legs to a 90-degree angle, or as high as you can with proper form.

3. Once you have reached the top position, reverse the movement to complete one repetition.

NB: Avoid touching your feet on the ground at the end of each rep. Maintaining core tension is key to building strength and stability.

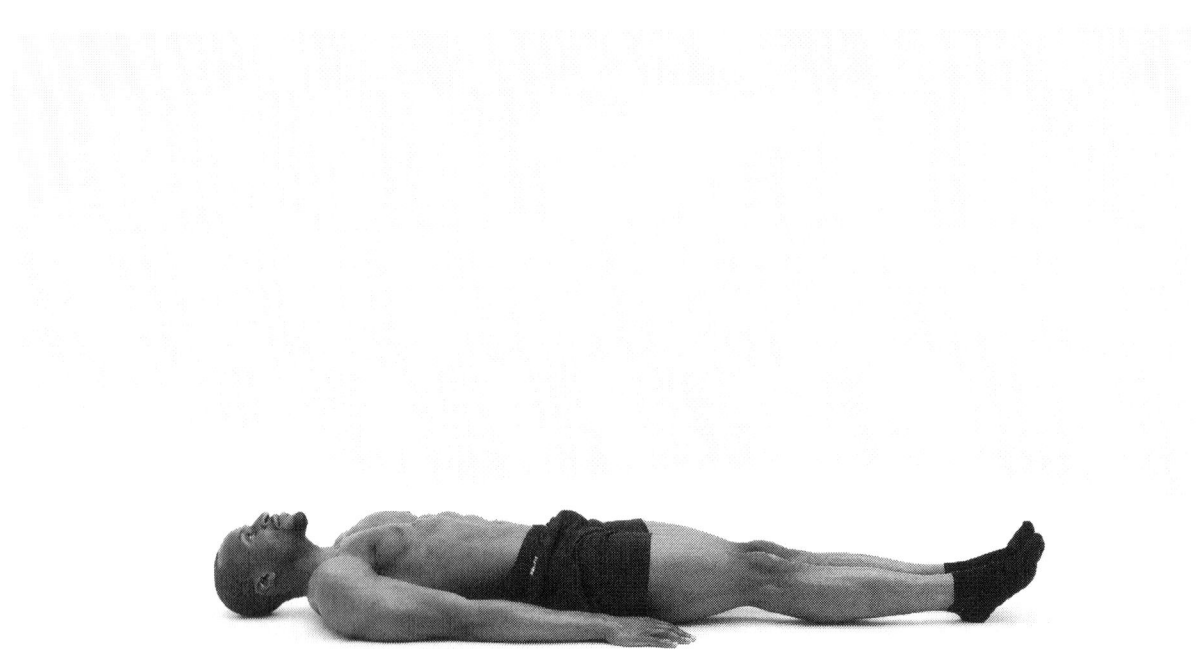

Fundamentals

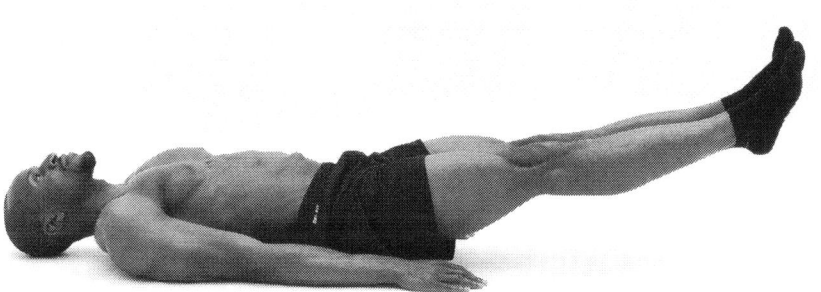

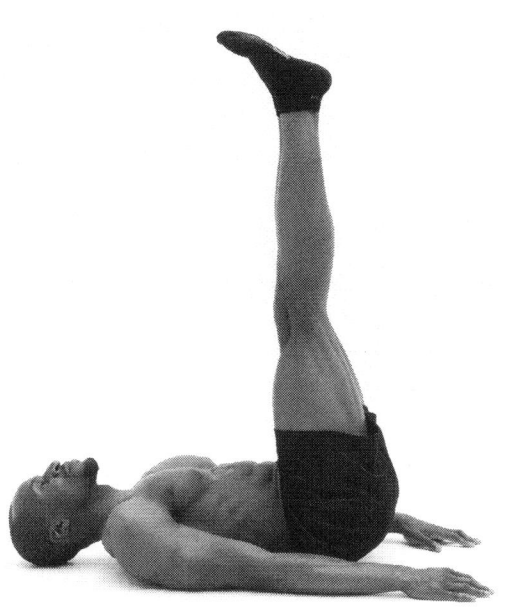

Rear Arch

You will work your lower back with almost every core exercise you perform, but this is the first one we will cover which actually targets this area specifically.

Perform: 3-4 sets of 8-10 second hold times.

1. Lie down on your front and place your fingertips against your temples just as you did during sit-ups.

2. Aiming to keep your hips rooted to the floor, contract the muscles in your lower back and raise both your head and feet up as if you were trying to make them meet behind your back.

3. Hold for allotted time and then return to starting position to complete one rep.

Variations:

• When you have achieved your set / hold time gradually increase the hold time to keep improving.

• Try extending your arms out straight in front to make the exercise more difficult.

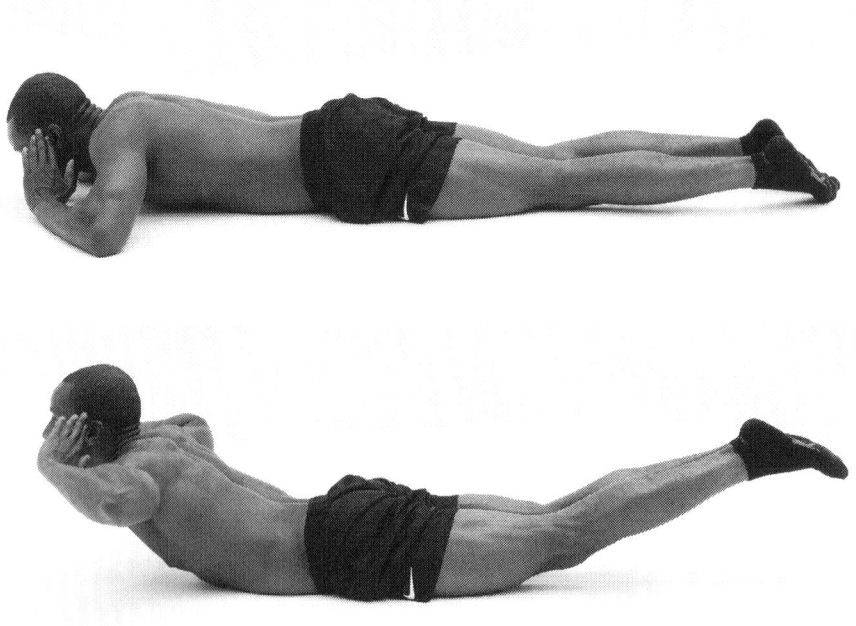

Fundamentals

REAR SUPPORT

This one will really engage your core muscles while opening up your hip flexors to help you perform the lower body stuff to come.

Perform: 3-4 sets of 10-15 second hold times.

1. Sit on the ground with your legs straight out in front of you and your hands by your sides, fingers facing backwards.

2. Balancing on your hands and heels, push your hips up and try to align your whole body from ankles to shoulders.

3. Hold this position for as long as possible to complete one set. As with all such exercises, gradually increase the hold time to improve your strength and resistance.

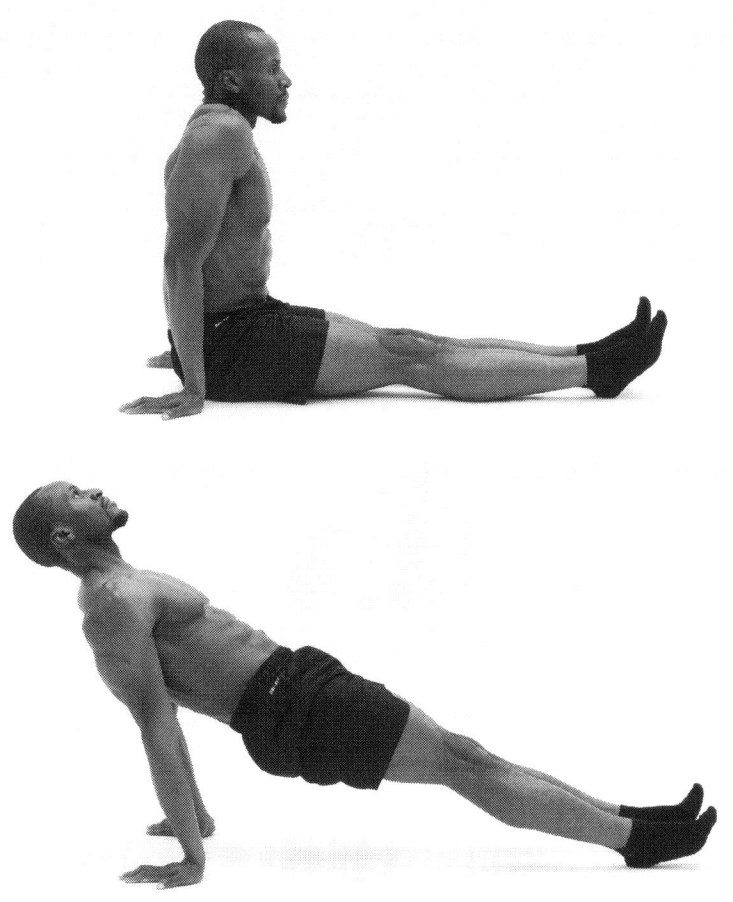

KNEE RAISES

Once you are comfortable with floor core exercises, head on over to a dip station or pull-up bar for a different kind of challenge.

Perform: 3-4 sets of 15-20 reps.

You will need: dip station / pull-up bar.

1. Grab the bar with an overhand grip and hang freely.

2. Bend your knees and draw your legs up towards your chest, contracting your core hard and focusing all the tension on the target muscles.

3. Return your legs to the starting position to complete one repetition. Make sure you are using your core and not momentum to achieve this movement.

Variation: If you don't have access to the equipment shown, you can use a dip station or captain's chair instead.

NB: It's not just your core that can tire during exercises like this. You might find your grip giving out, or your thighs burning up, for example.

This is your body's way of telling you that you have weak links somewhere in the chain. The good news is that with calisthenics you are almost always working more than one muscle group.

So, you will find that while you are doing knee raises to build a strong core, you are also generating forearm gains or hip flexibility, among other things.

Just don't forget that proper form is everything; if another area of your body is holding you back, make a note to work harder on that instead of cheating your way through.

Fundamentals

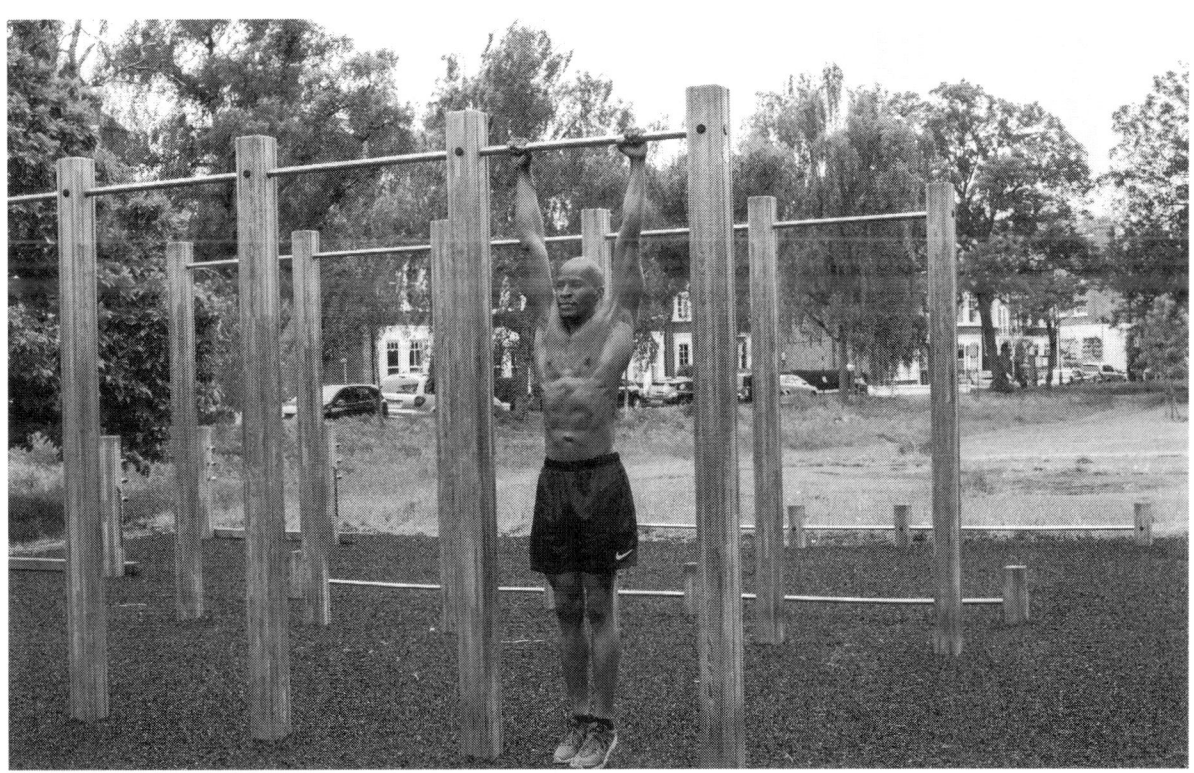

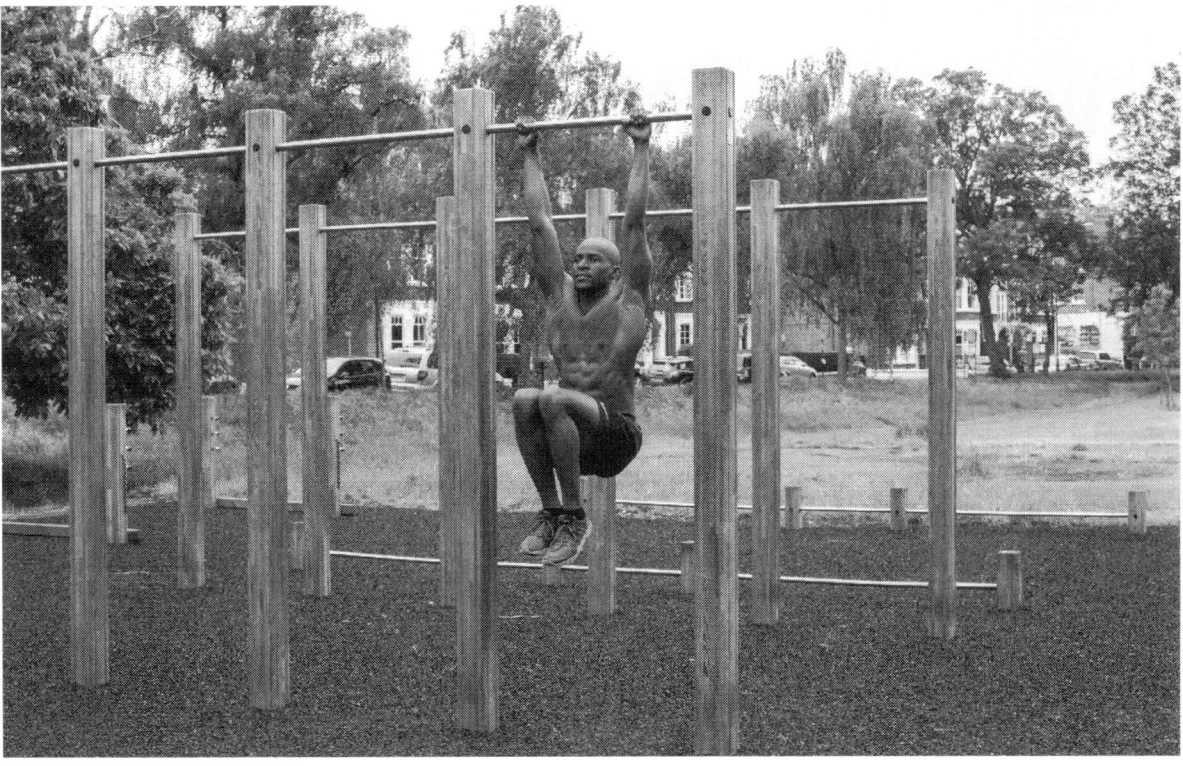

5. Exercises - Core

LEG RAISES

The natural progression from knee raises is to keep your legs straight and perform a similar movement, reaching up as high as you can without sacrificing form.

Perform: 3-4 sets of 10-15 reps.

You will need: a pull-up bar.

1. Grasp the bar with an overhand grip and let your legs hang straight down.

2. Using your core and not momentum, aim to bring your feet all the way up to your hands, keeping your legs straight throughout the movement.

3. Bring your legs back down to the start position to complete one rep.

NB: If you can't complete this range of movement, simply raise your legs as high as possible and increase the distance over time. The goal is to use your core for the vast majority of the movement, so do not lean back to achieve this until you are right at the top. Start by trying to get your legs parallel to the ground without moving your upper body.

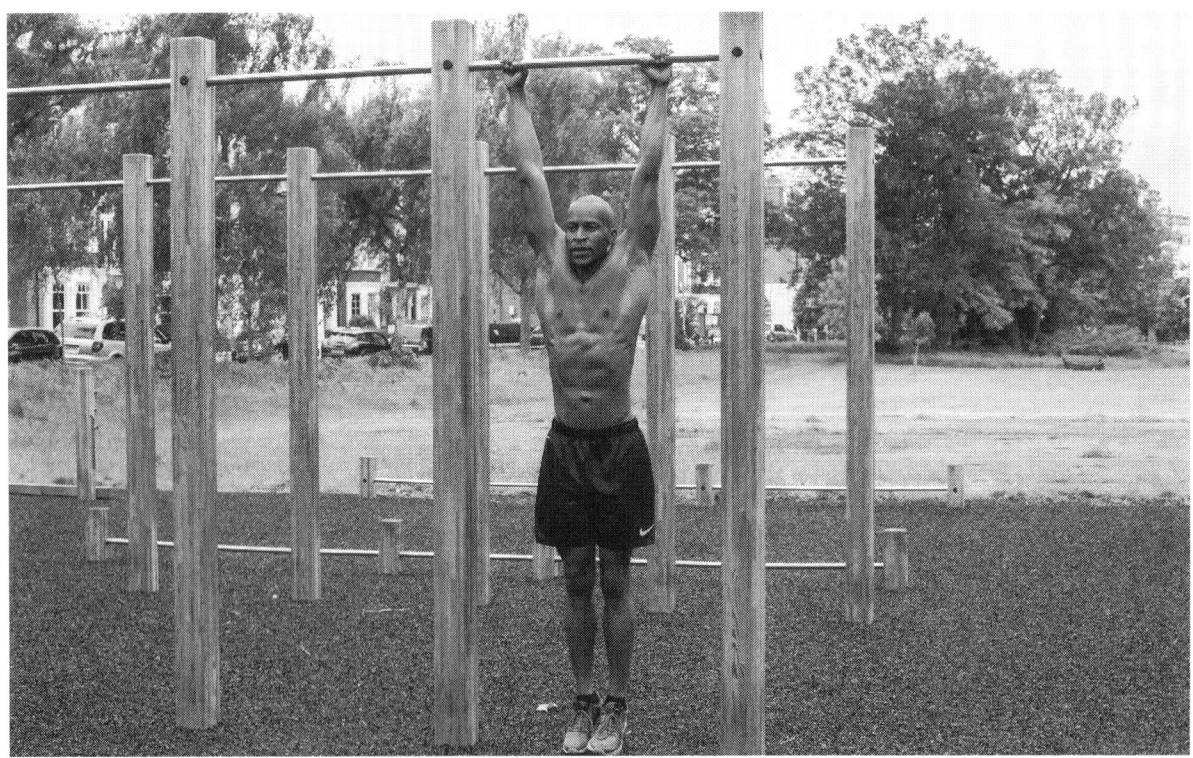

Fundamentals

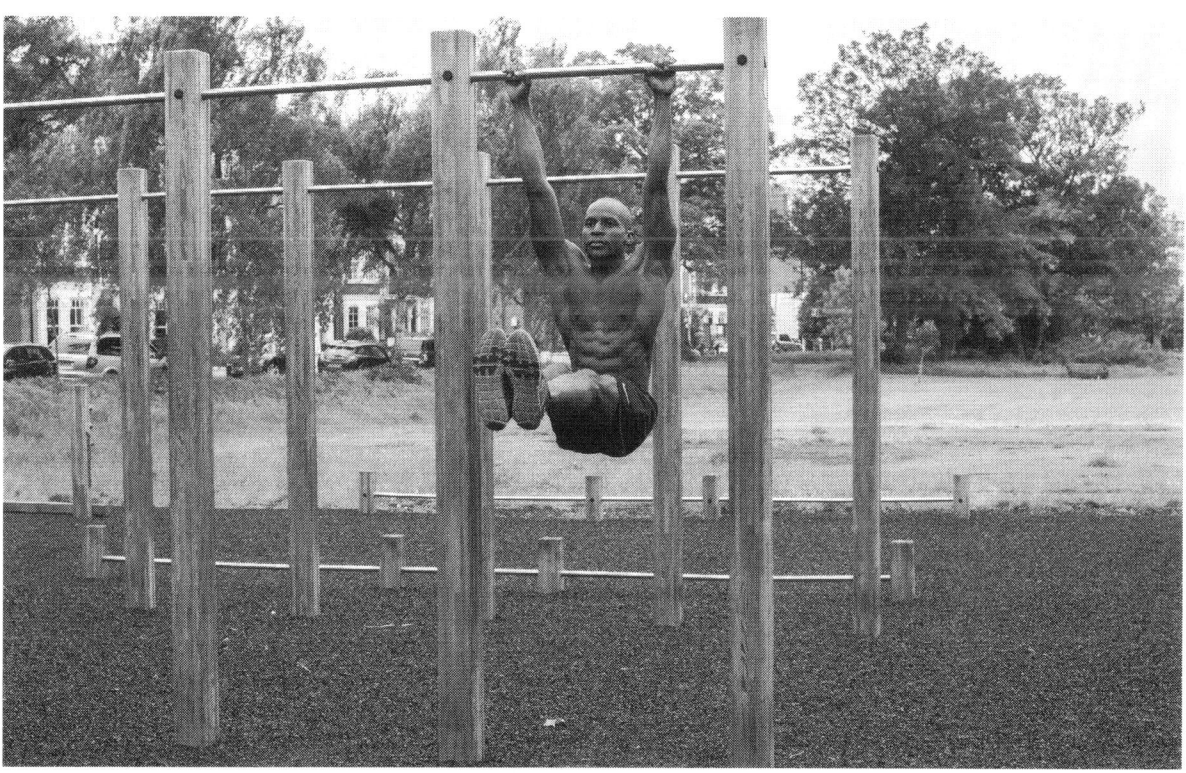

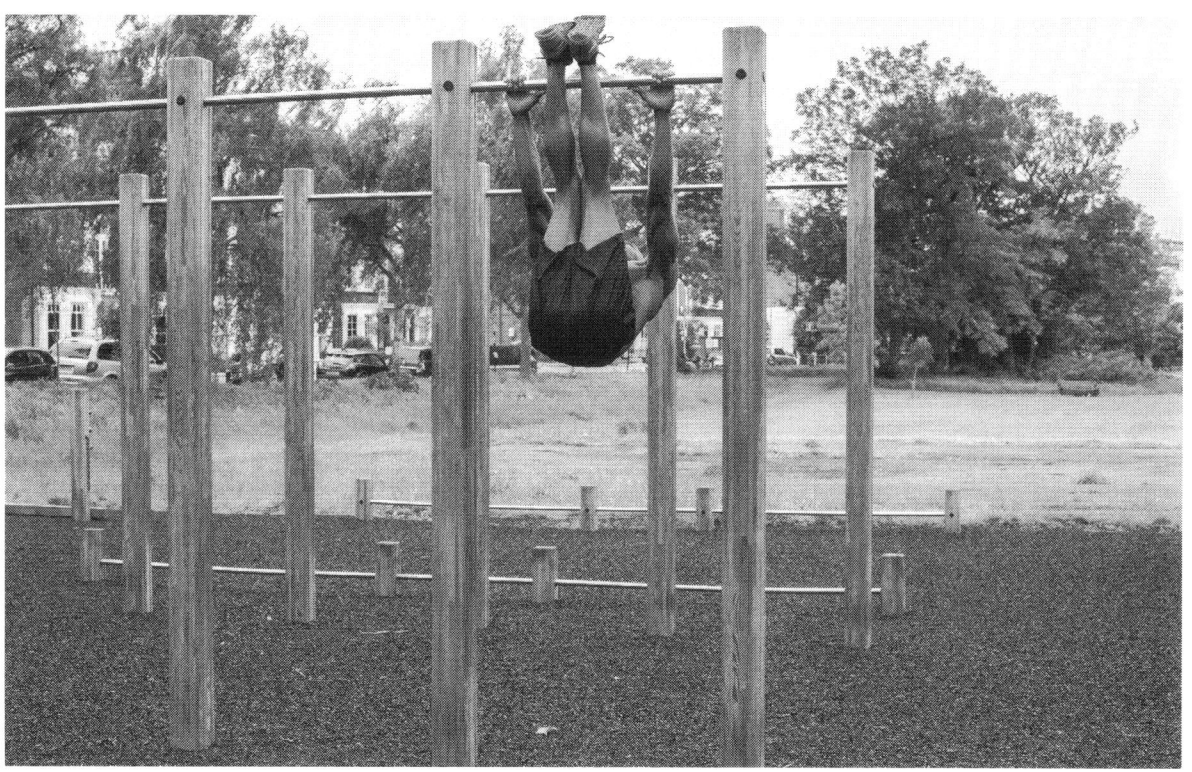

5. Exercises - Core

WINDOW WIPERS

These little gems will burn out your core very quickly, but keep at them! They are an incredibly effective abs, obliques and lower back building exercise.

Perform: 3-4 sets of 6-10 reps.

You will need: pull-up bar.

1. Assume a standard overhand grip on the bar and hang freely.

2. Now raise your legs up until your toes or shins are touching the bar. Remember to keep your arms and legs straight.

3. Now move your legs all the way to one side as far as you can. Think of your legs as windshield wipers going back and forth.

4. Once you reach your flexibility limit on one side. Reverse the direction and take your legs all the way to the other side. This counts as 1 rep.

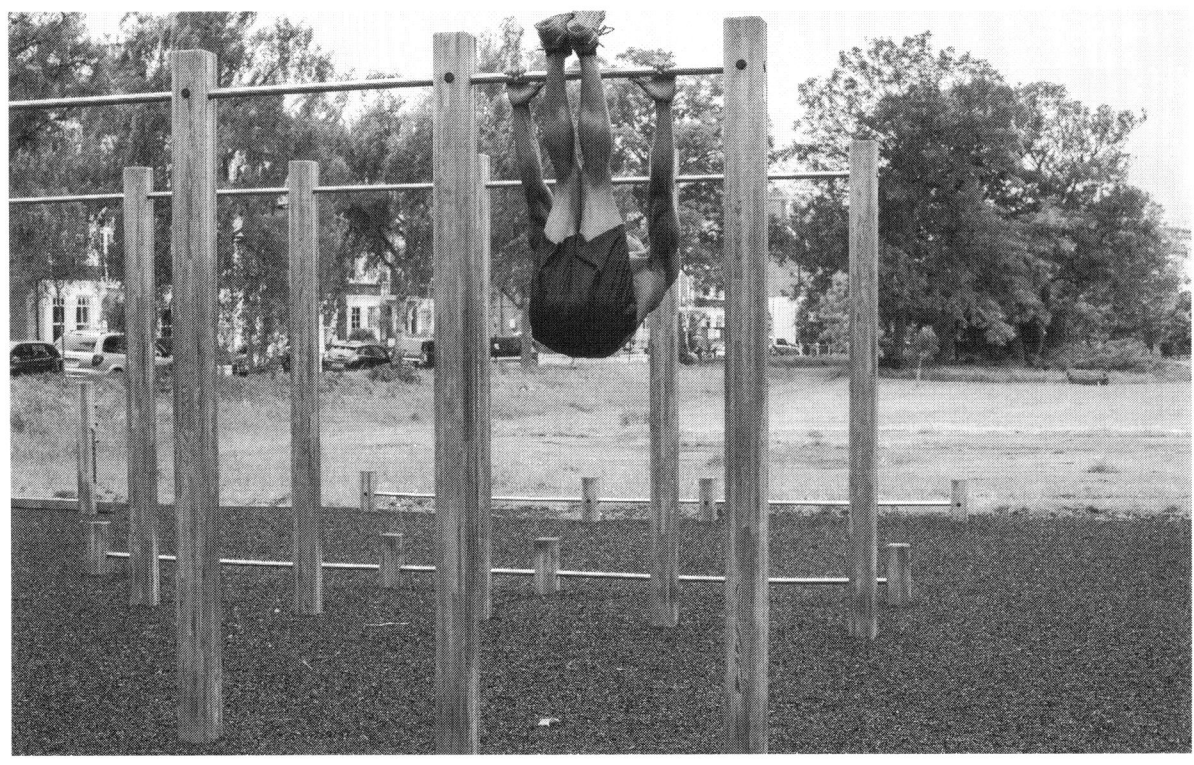

Fundamentals

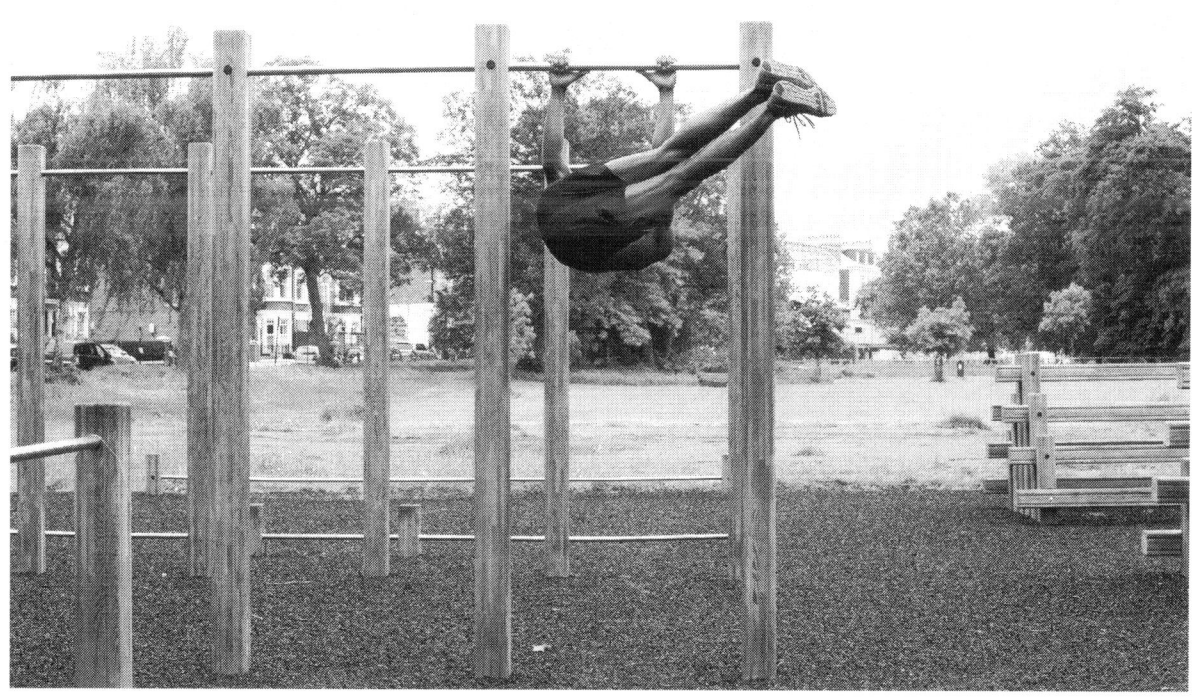

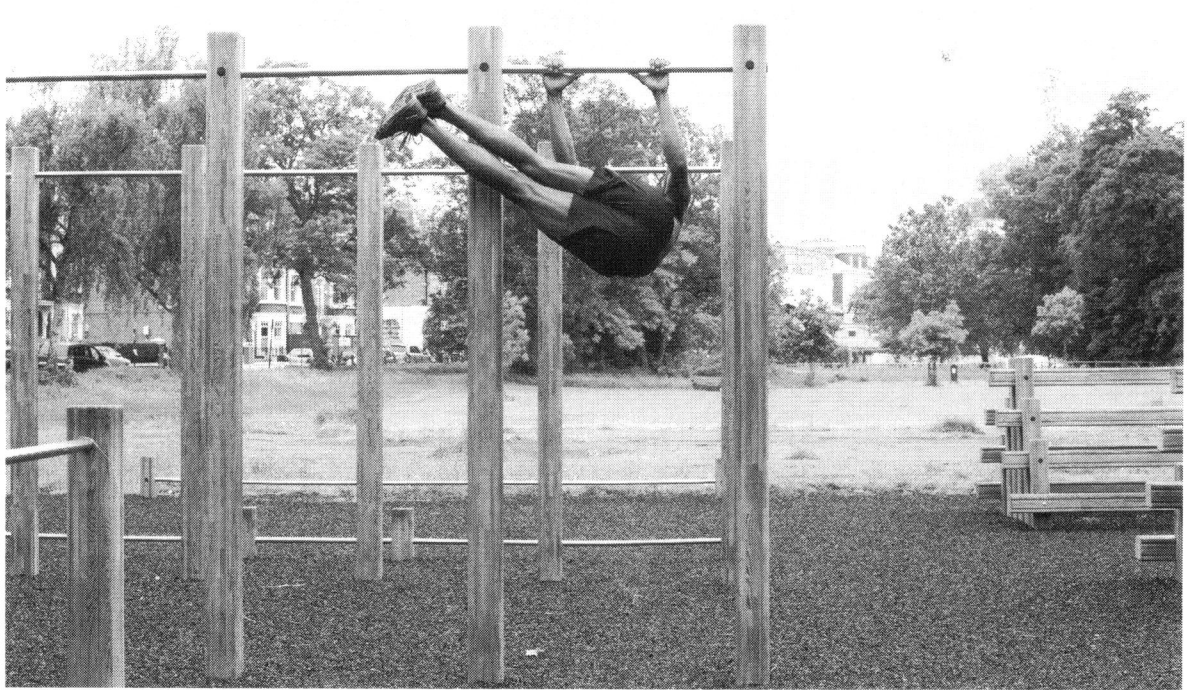

Dragon Flag

It will take several steps to master this core crusher, but stick at it and you will benefit from insane results. Remember, it is better to master the fundamentals with proper form than to rush ahead and do things incorrectly. Without further ado, let's get to it!

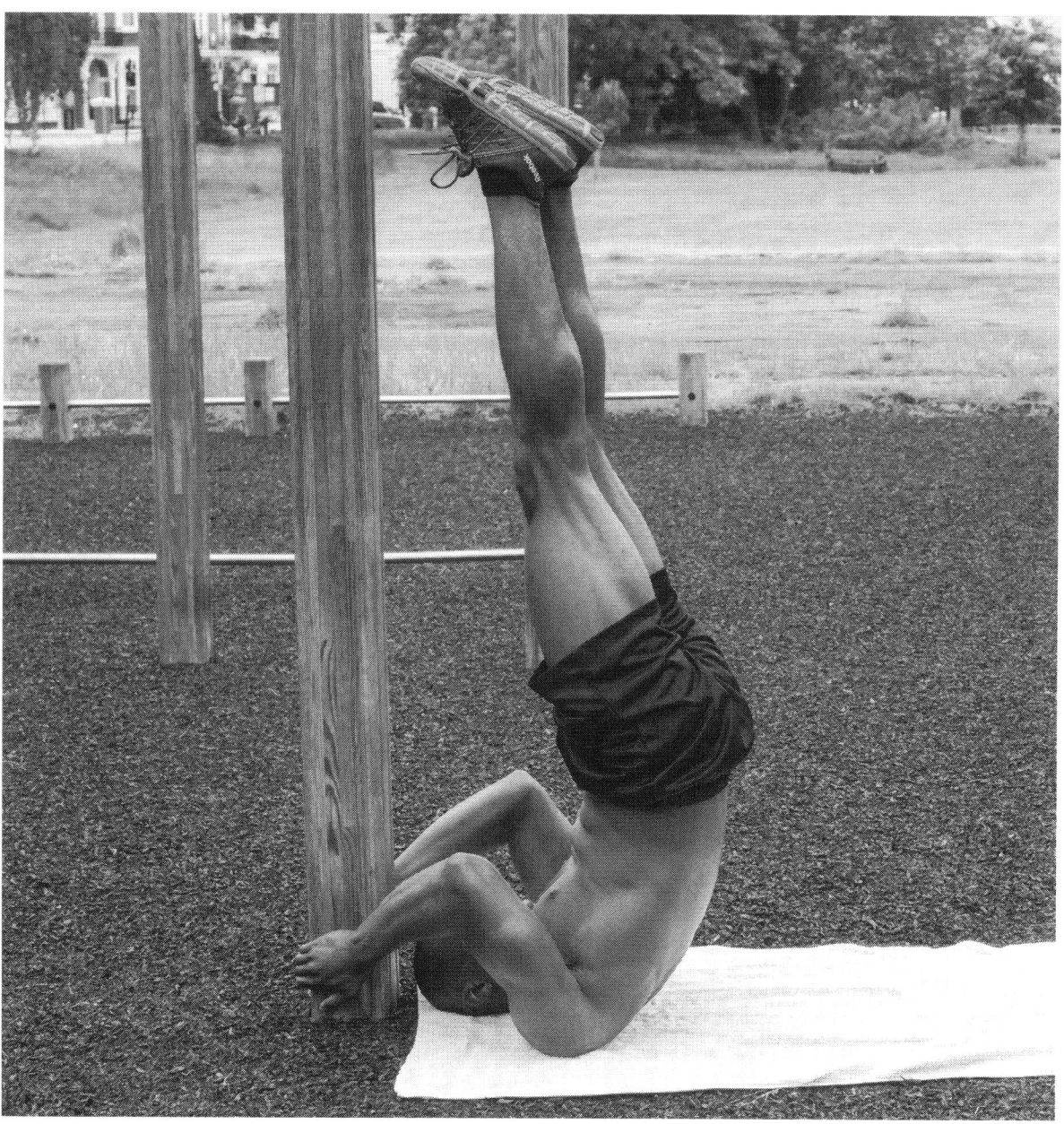

5. Exercises - Core

CANDLESTICK POSITION

As you embark on your quest to conquer the dragon flag, an excellent starting point is to become comfortable with the candlestick.

Get accustomed to using your shoulders to support your bodyweight, and work on range of motion so you can achieve this position without straining your shoulders or neck.

Perform: 3-4 sets of 15-20 second hold times.

You will need: strong vertical bar or post and a bench or platform if you wish. Neck cushioning also recommended.

1. Lie on your back with your feet pointing away from the post, your head a few inches away, grasping the post behind you.

2. Now engage your core and pull your legs into your chest, then raise yourself onto your shoulders.

3. Extend your legs straight up and point your toes. Your body should be vertical from shoulders to toes.

4. Hold for as long as possible.

Variation: You can also perform this exercise lying on a bench that is placed around a foot from the post, horizontally aligned.

This will give your head enough room to dip comfortably over the edge. In this case, it is essential to use a sturdy bench and a spotter to ensure everything is stable.

Dragon Flag

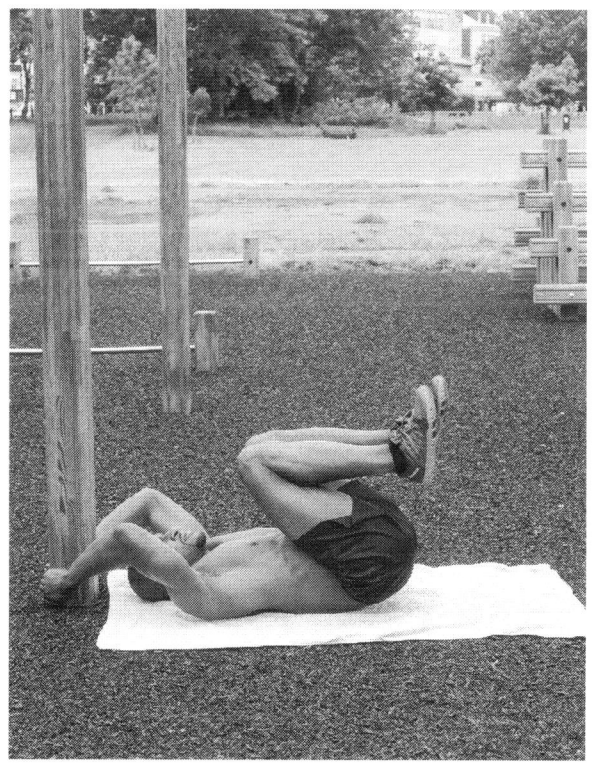
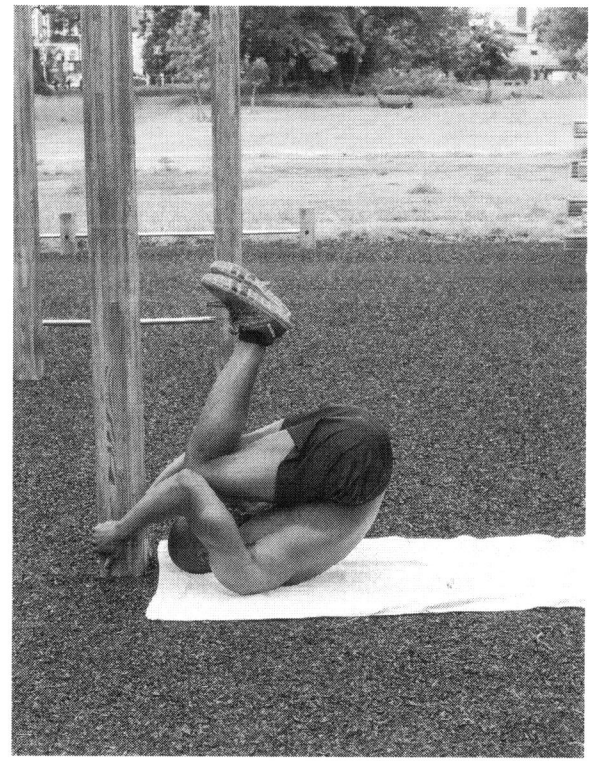
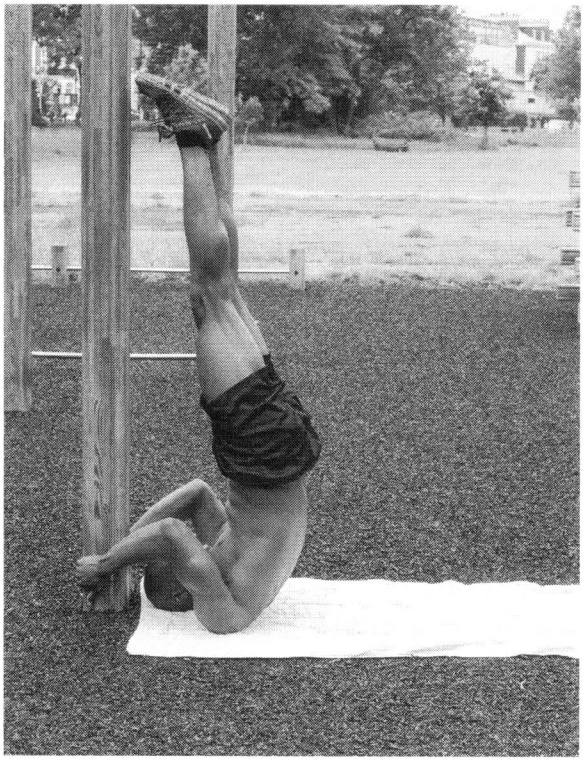

TUCK DRAGON FLAG

Once you are comfortable supporting your weight on your shoulders, it's time to move on to the dynamic movement of the dragon flag. We'll start with the tucked version, and work on extending those legs later.

Perform: 3-4 sets of 6-8 reps.

You will need: strong vertical bar or post and a bench or platform if you wish.

1. Assume the same starting position as the candlestick, flat on your back, grasping the post behind you.

2. Pull your knees into your chest, and raise your torso up onto your shoulders.

3. Continue to raise your torso and pivot on your shoulders until your knees are almost touching your face and the bottoms of your feet are facing straight up, or as high as you can get them.

4. Now slowly lower yourself back to the starting position. This counts as 1 rep. Practice gently rolling back and forth in preparation for extending your legs later.

Super important: Using momentum or forcing your bodyweight back onto your neck is dangerous and will not result in any progress.

When rolling back, focus the strain in your core and ensure you have a firm grip on the fixture. This should be enough to achieve the position with proper form. If not, just do what you can and keep building up to it.

Dragon Flag

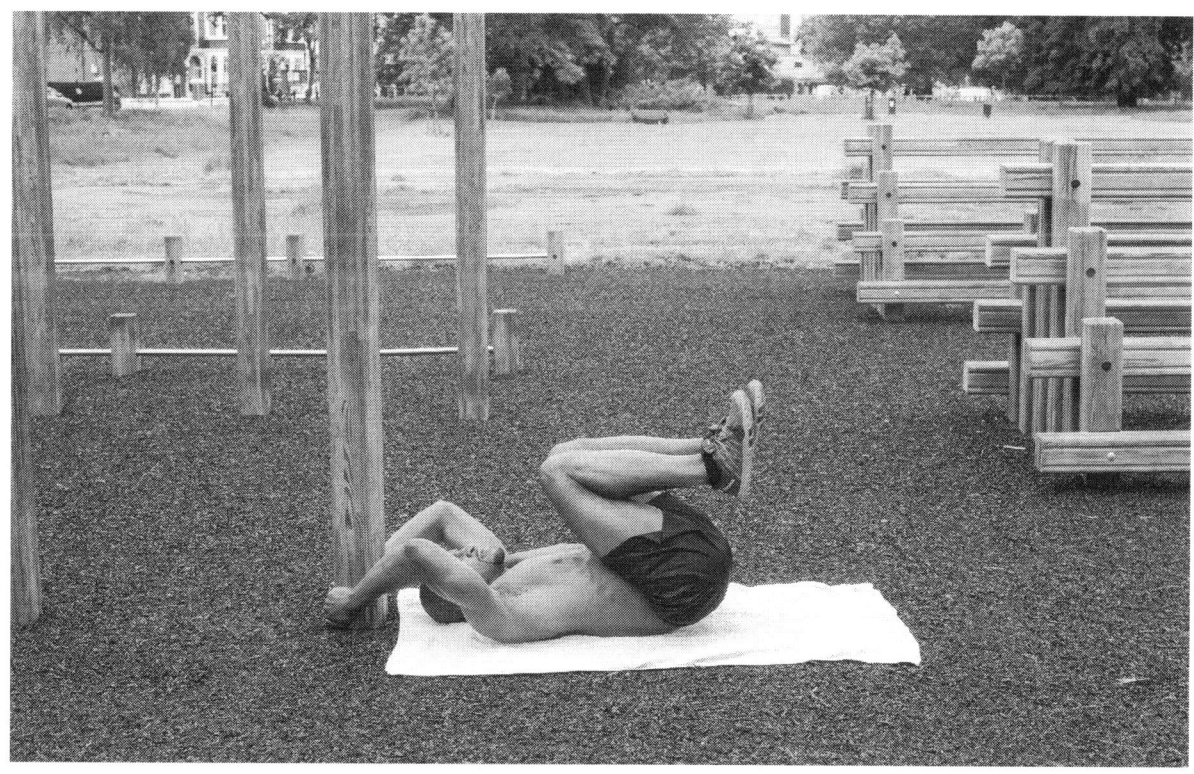

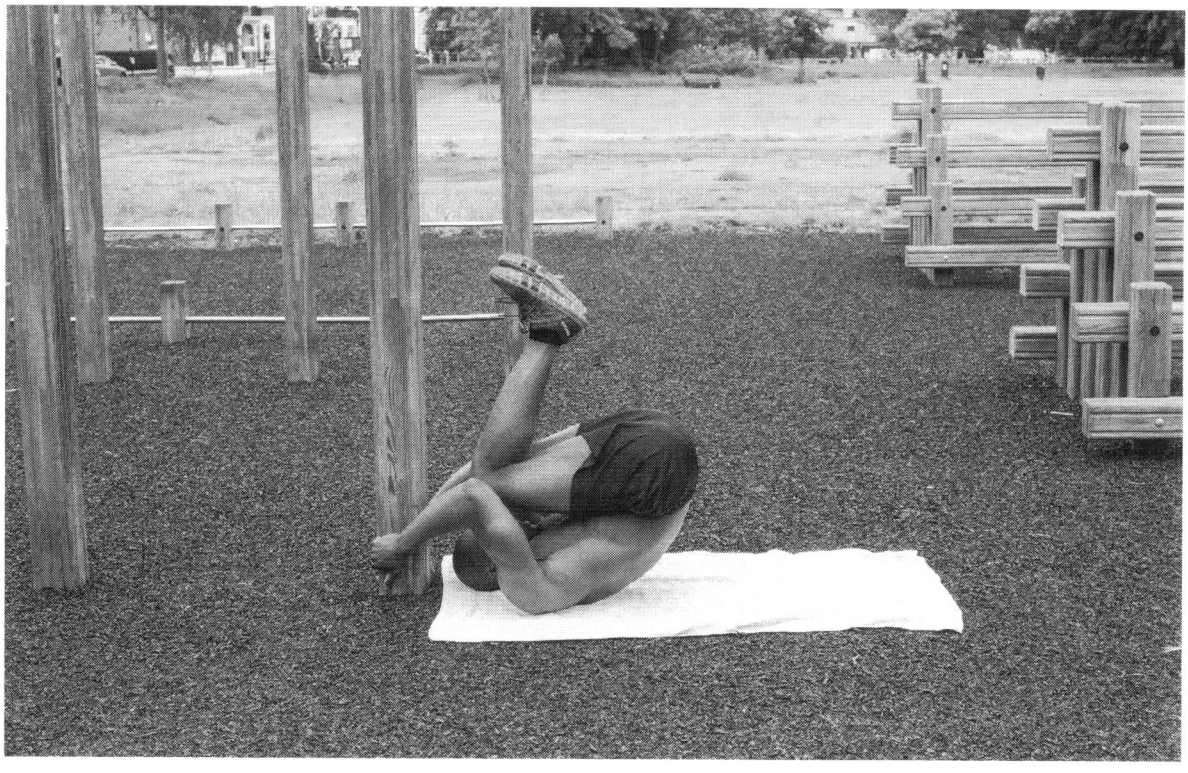

SINGLE-LEG EXTENSION DRAGON FLAG

Now that you are comfortable with the motion associated with the dragon flag. We'll move on to extending one leg for an increased challenge. Remember to alternate legs between sets for an even workout!

Perform: 3-4 sets of 3-6 reps.

You will need: strong vertical bar or post and a bench if you wish.

1. Assume the candlestick position described before, grasping the bar behind your head, as vertical as you can get.

2. Now retract one leg and pull it into your chest while keeping the other completely locked out.

3. Slowly lower yourself to the floor by pivoting on your shoulders. Remember to keep your core rigid.

4. Once you touch the floor, raise yourself back to the starting position. This counts as a single rep. Tough, right?

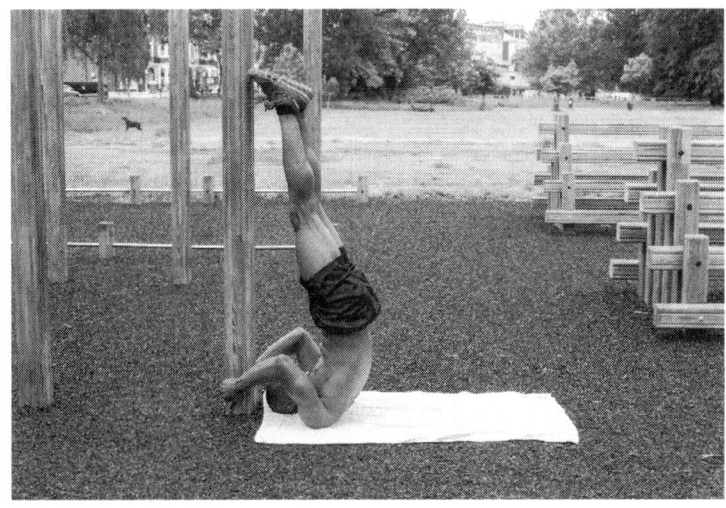

Dragon Flag

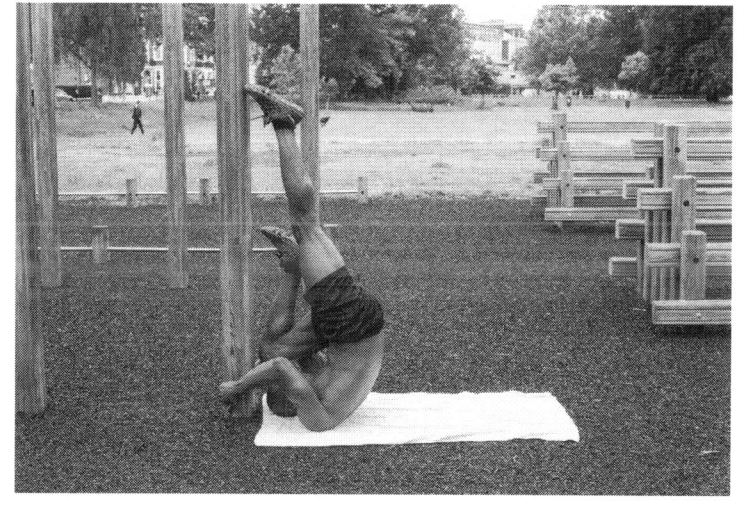

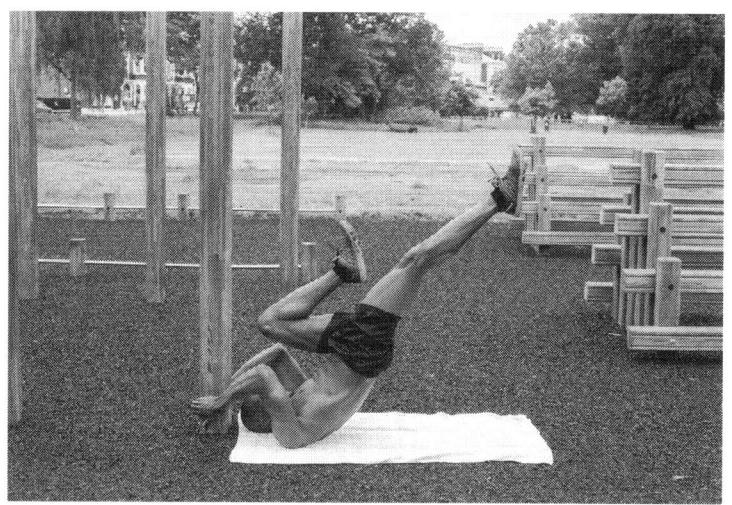

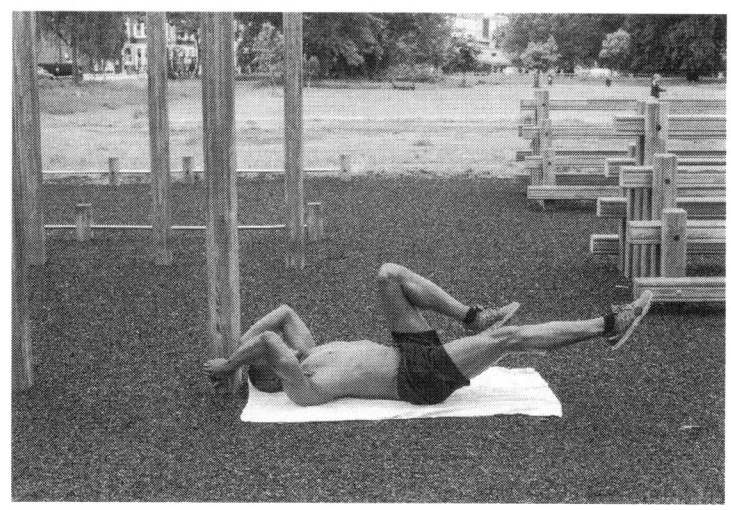

5. Exercises - Core

NEGATIVE DRAGON FLAG

Before we jump into the full dragon flag we're first going to complete some negative repetitions. This simply means that we'll start at the top of the movement, and slowly lower ourselves back down to get used to the strain and movement.

Perform: 3-4 sets of 3-6 reps.

You will need: strong vertical bar or post and a bench if you wish.

1. Assume the candlestick position.

2. Slowly lower yourself to the ground by pivoting at the shoulders. Always remember, we want to keep a straight line from shoulders to toes so don't bend at the core!

3. Once you reach the ground, or as low as you can go, this counts as a single repetition. Reset to the candlestick and repeat.

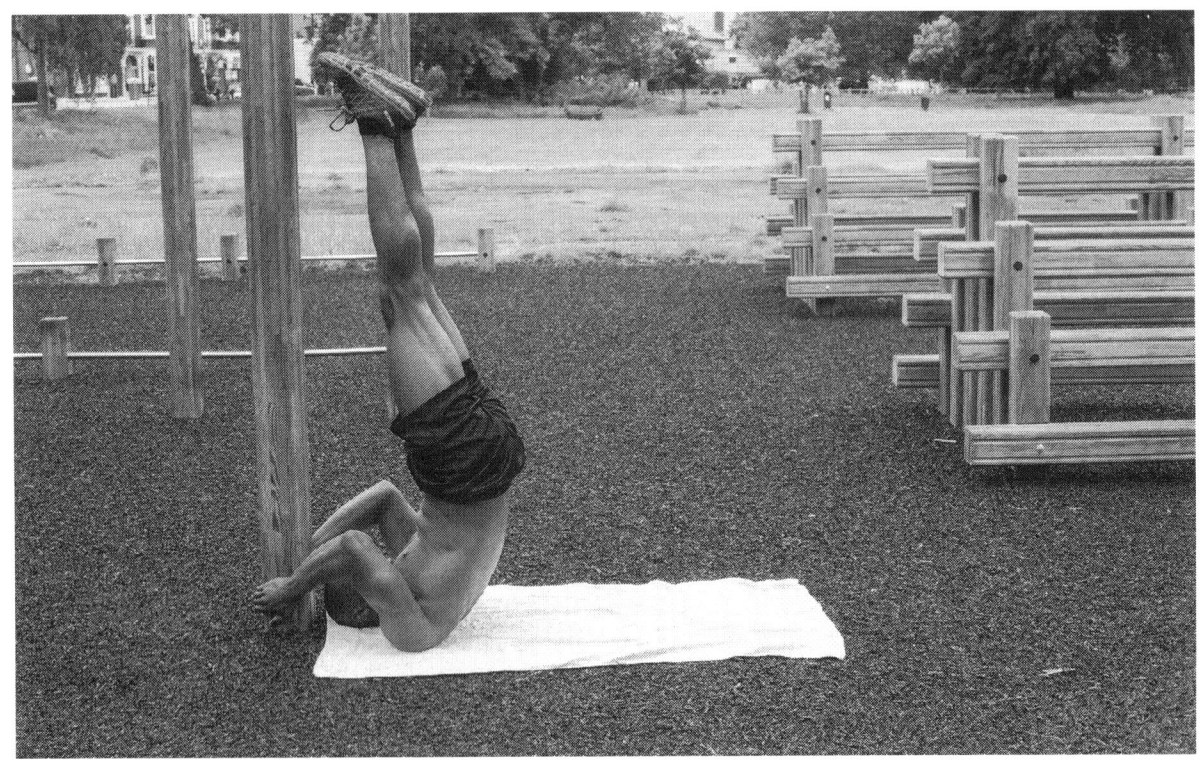

Dragon Flag

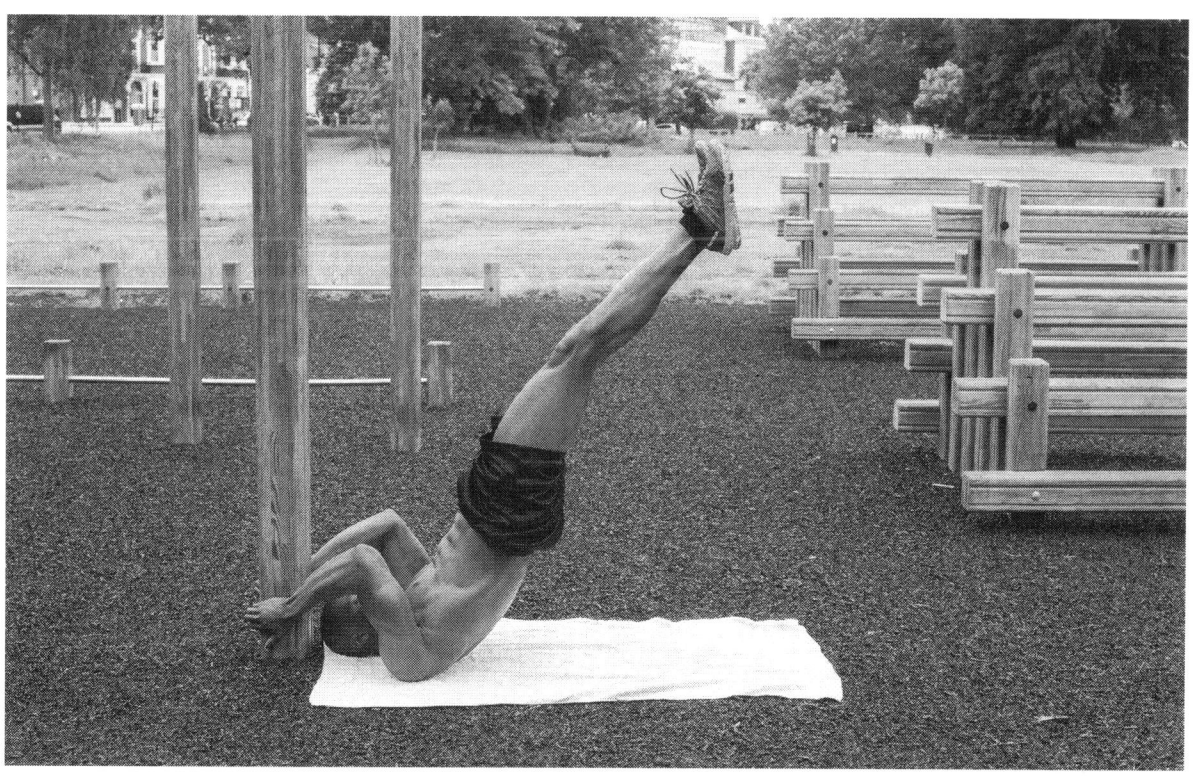

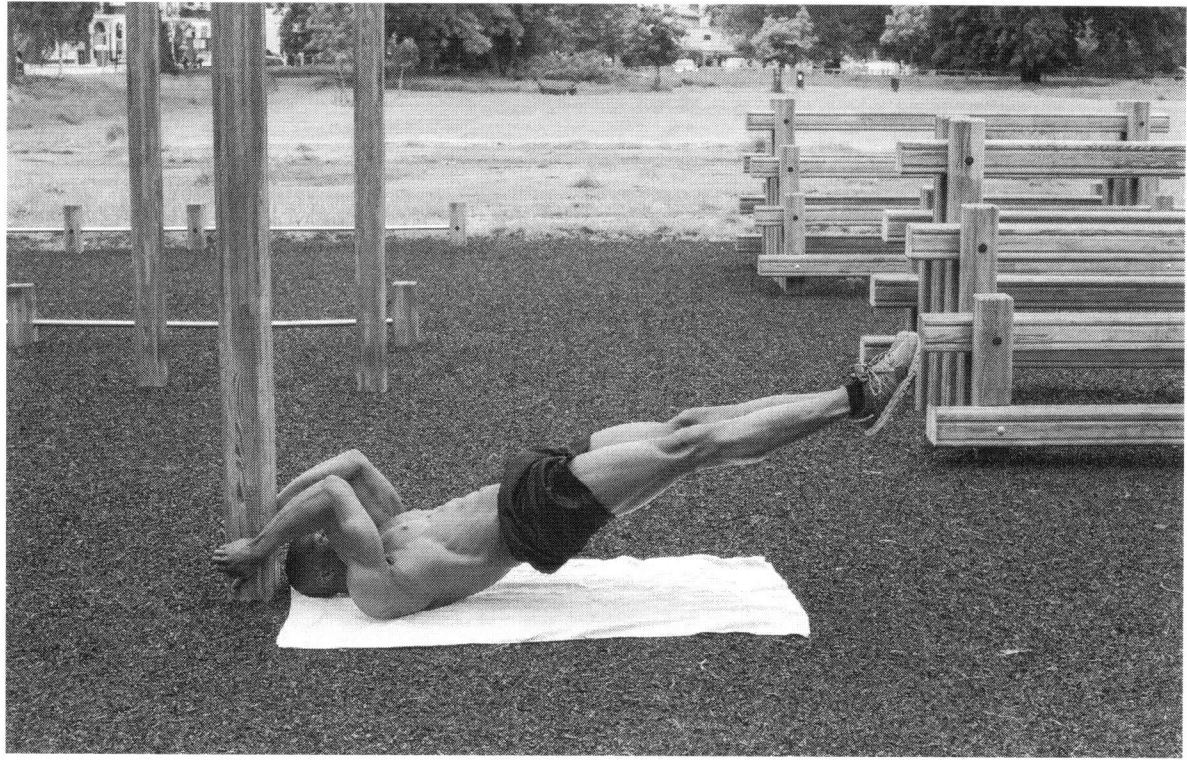

COMPLETE DRAGON FLAG

When you are comfortable with the negative dragon flag movements, we can move on to the full dragon flag.

This is achieved by raising yourself back up to a vertical position, while maintaining a straight body, without having to reset to the candlestick.

Perform: 3-4 sets of 3-6 reps.

You will need: strong vertical bar or post and a bench or platform if you wish.

1. Assume the candlestick position.

2. Now lower yourself just as you would for the negative dragon flag. Remember to keep your body straight from shoulders to toes! This will get easier with time.

3. Once you reach the ground, immediately reverse the motion and pull yourself back up to the starting position. Congrats, that's a rep!

Super important: This is an immensely difficult exercise, so it's worth mentioning again that true form is everything, and you should never cheat your way through sets.

When dealing with sensitive areas such as the neck, it is absolutely essential that you don't try to perform anything you are not comfortable with.

As always, if you are finding it too difficult, flick back a through pages and master the simpler variations before moving on.

Dragon Flag

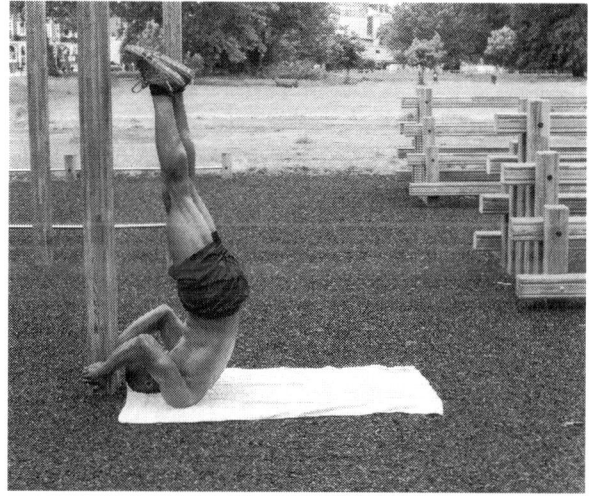
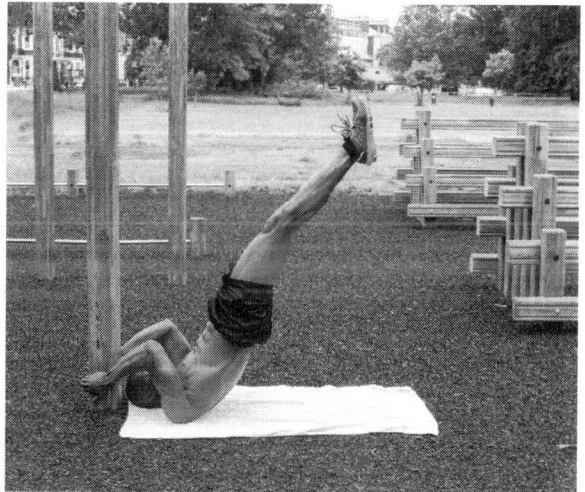
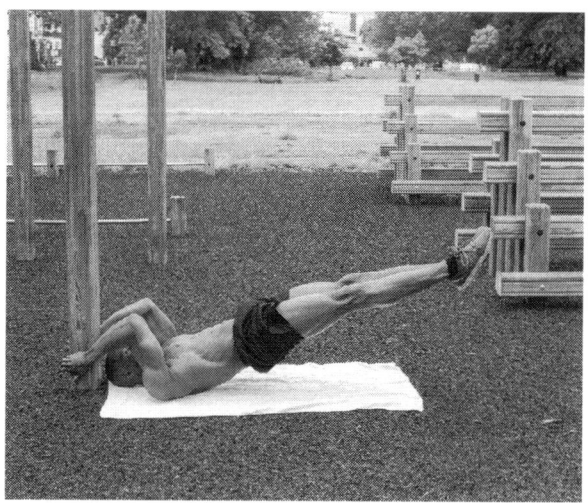
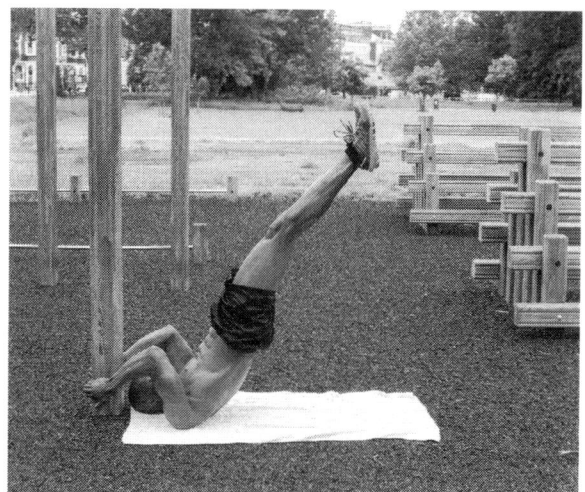
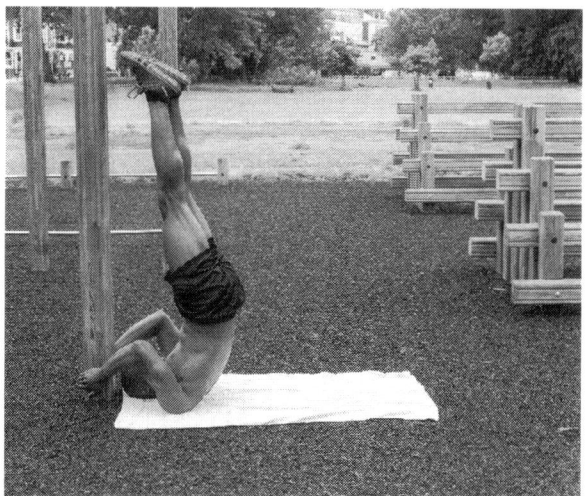

DRAGON FLAG KICKS

To make the dragon flag a little more challenging, throw in some leg movement. This will be extremely taxing on your core, but the additional motion is extremely beneficial.

Perform: 2-3 sets of 15-20 seconds worth.

You will need: strong vertical bar or post and a bench or platform if you wish.

1. Assume the candlestick position.

2. Now slowly lower yourself as you would for a dragon flag, stopping with your feet slightly above the ground.

3. Once you are in position move your legs up and down in a controlled motion, much like you would during a gentle swim.

4. Continue for as long as you are able, then take a quick rest, reset to the candlestick position and repeat.

Variations:

• Perform single leg extensions by drawing one leg up towards your chest while keeping the other extended, and then switching.

• Mix it up with a continuous 'cycling' motion. Just remember to focus the strain in your core and never on your neck.

If you've just pulled of a full 3 sets of 20 seconds, then congratulations, you've mastered the dragon flag series!

Your core should be growing accustomed to the stresses and strains of calisthenics, and you will need every ounce of experience gained to take on our next group of exercises.

Grab the parallettes, it's time to take on another bodyweight exercise icon.

Dragon Flag

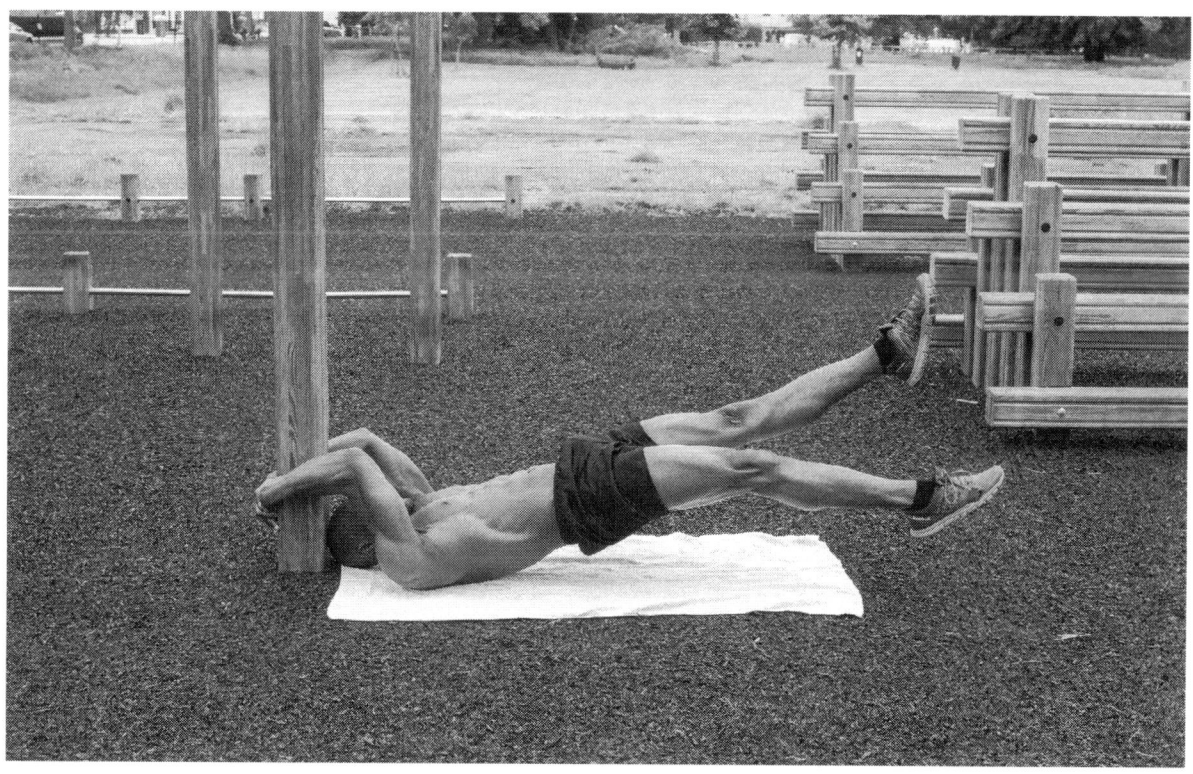

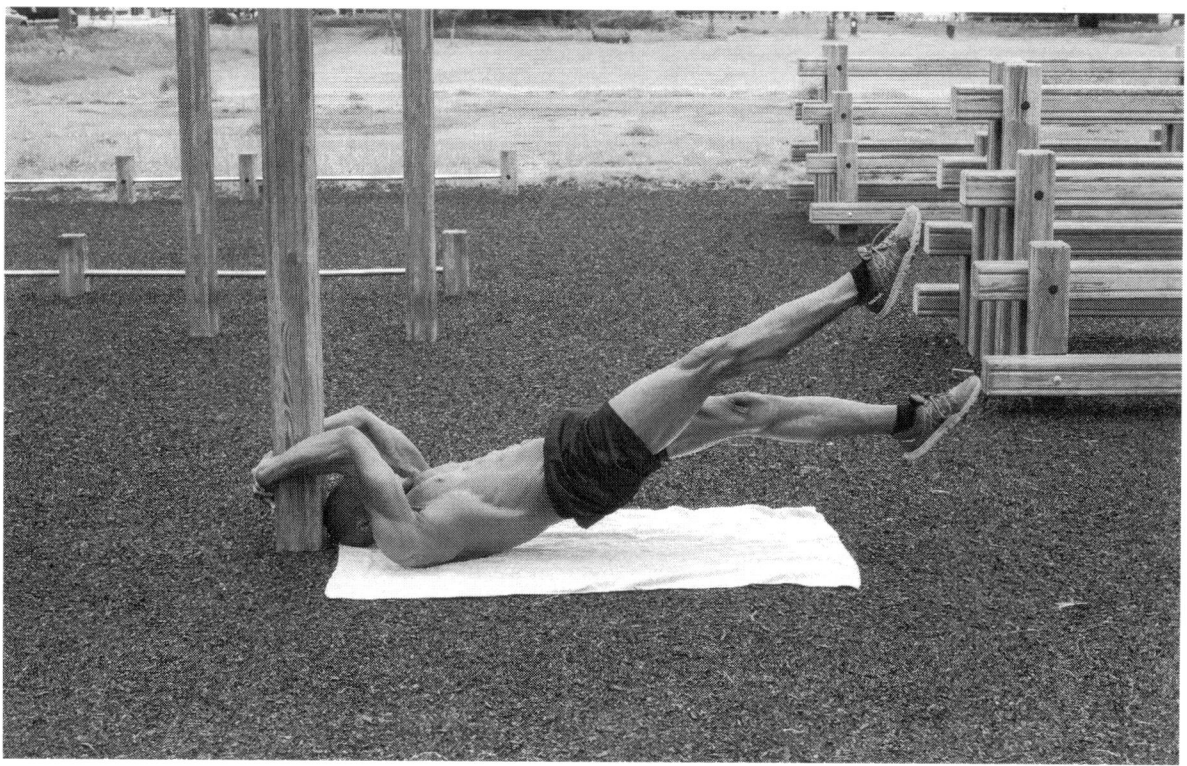

HALF LEVER

The half lever will get that six-pack popping while simultaneously strengthening your arms, legs and grip. We'll be using parallettes and, as you have probably come to expect, we'll start with the tucked position and build up to the full version from there. Vamos!

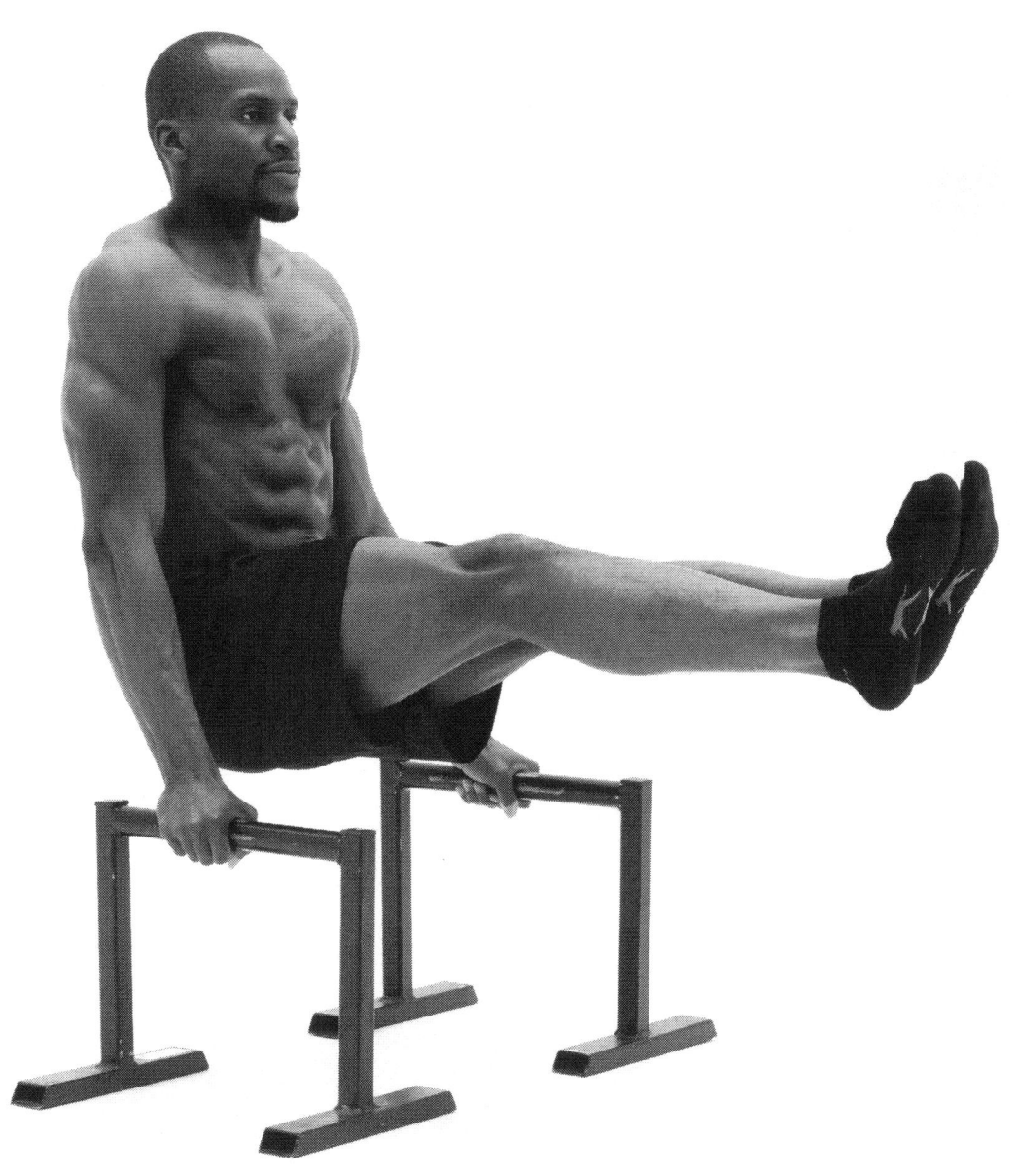

TUCK HALF LEVER

If you're all warmed up we'll get started with the basic tucked version of this exercise in order to introduce the concept and build core strength. We'll move on to more difficult positions in the following exercises.

Perform: 20-30 second hold time.

You will need: parallettes or two other sturdy, raised platforms.

1. Position yourself between the parallettes, grasp them, and push yourself up. Your hands and elbows should be directly under your shoulders and in line with your hips.

2. Now engage your core and keep your knees bent at 90 degrees. Lift your legs until your thighs are at 90 degrees to your torso, or horizontal.

3. Hold for long as possible.

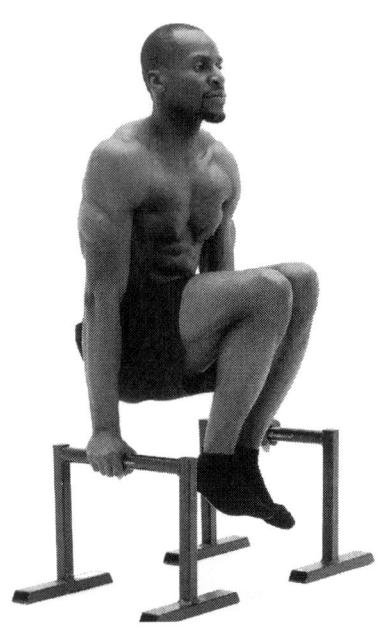

Half Lever

PARTIAL HALF LEVER

This will be exactly the same position as the tucked lever, except we'll extend the legs slightly to put a little more strain on your core. Remember to keep your elbows locked out for the entire hold time.

Perform: 20-30 second hold time.

You will need: parallettes or two other sturdy, raised platforms.

1. Assume the tucked half lever that we already introduced.

2. Once you are in position, with locked out arms, extend your legs until they are about half way to being straight.

3. Hold for as long as possible.

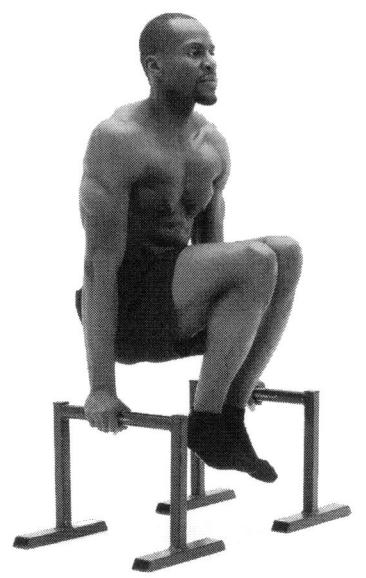
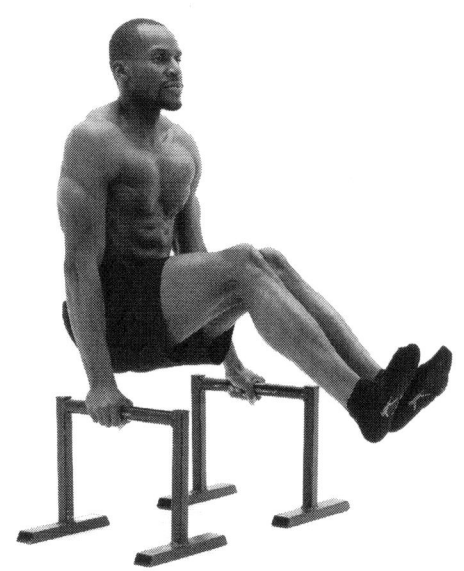

Complete Half Lever

When you are comfortable with the partial half lever, move on to the complete version. Remember to maintain rigidity throughout your entire body and control your breathing in order to control your posture.

Perform: 20-30 second hold time.

You will need: parallettes or two other sturdy, raised platforms.

1. Take up the tuck or partial half lever.

2. Now extend your legs to their full extent out in front of you. Lock out your knees!

3. Hold for as long as possible and try not to mess yourself.

Variation: Remove the parallettes and use the floor instead for a greater challenge. This will reduce the amount of control you have to maintain balance, so splay out your fingers and experiment with different hand orientations to find the one that works for you.

Remember: as with all timed exercises, if you cannot complete it all in one go, split it into sets of smaller increments to achieve the full hold time.

Don't be alarmed if you tremble like a leaf when first making the transition from partial to complete here. This is a natural response when testing the weakest links in your body, and will settle down as you become stronger over time.

As an additional tip, it is worth mentioning that the higher the parallettes, the easier the transition will be. If you have particularly low parallettes you may struggle due to the lack of ground clearance.

Half Lever

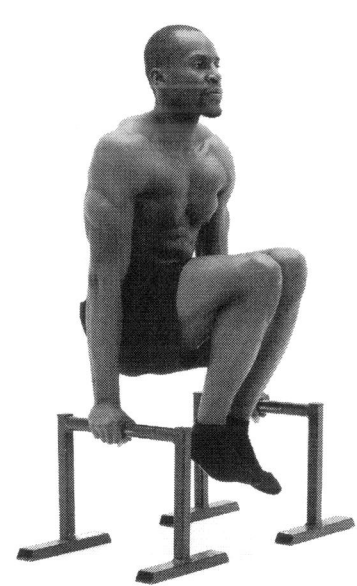
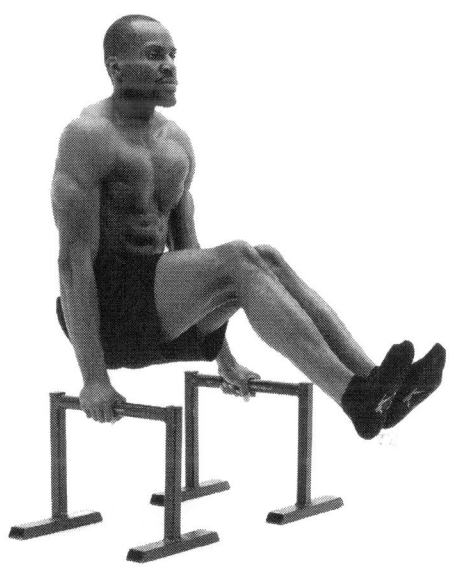
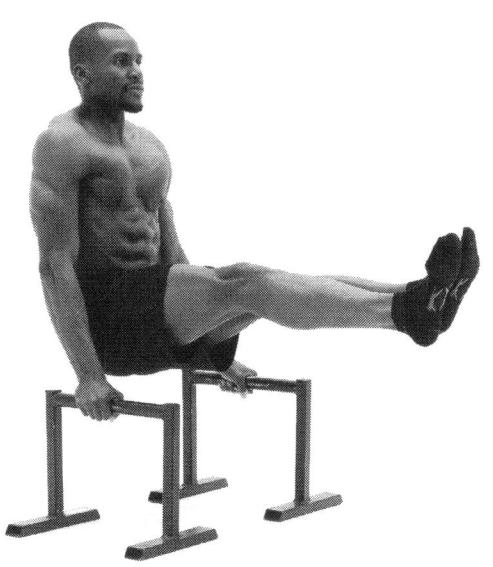

HALF LEVER LEG EXTENSIONS

Adding a little movement to the half lever will greatly increase your level of control in addition to building up your overall core strength.

In this case, we're essentially going to transition back and forth from the tuck half lever to the complete half lever.

Perform: 2-3 sets of 15-20 reps.

You will need: parallettes, if you wish.

1. Position yourself on the parallettes with your knees drawn up close to your chest, or as far as you can.

2. Now extend your legs and point your toes as you would for the full half lever.

3. Once your legs are completely locked out in front of you, retract them back to the starting position to complete a rep.

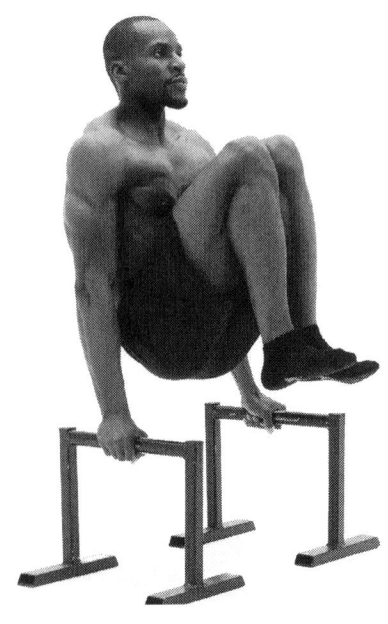

Half Lever

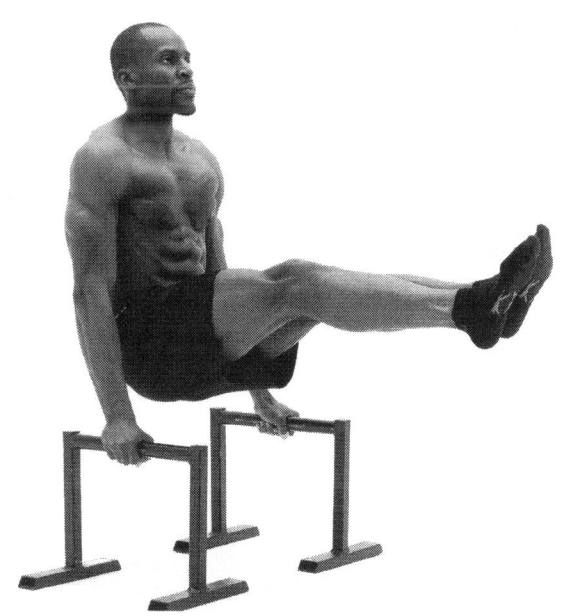

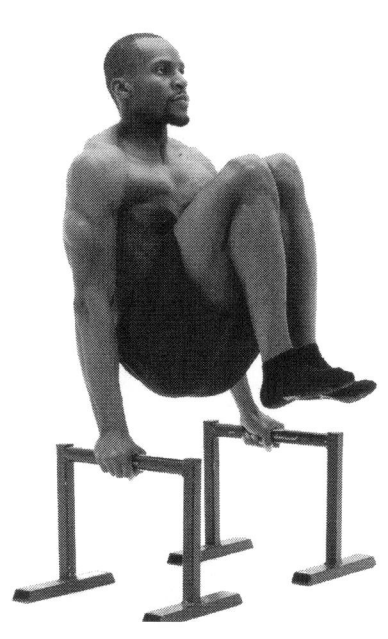

Half Lever Single Leg Extensions

Here we have subtle variation on the half lever leg extensions covered previously. While performing these, remember to keep your arms locked out and maintain your breathing level for as long as you can.

Perform: 20-30 seconds of non-stop reps.

You will need: parallettes, if you wish.

1. Assume the complete half lever position.

2. Now draw one knee towards your chest while keeping the other leg straight out in front of you.

3. Slowly bring the extended leg back in, and extend the other one straight out at the same time.

4. Repeat for allocated time.

Variations:

- Instead of sticking your legs straight out, perform the above in a 'cycling' motion.

- Keep both legs straight and kick them up and down as you did in dragon flag kicks.

If you are reading this fresh off your final set of half lever single leg extensions then you have officially passed this section with flying colors!

You have come through Core CRUSH like a champ, but it's not over yet. Next up we've got a healthy helping of cardio to finish things off with a bang!!

Half Lever

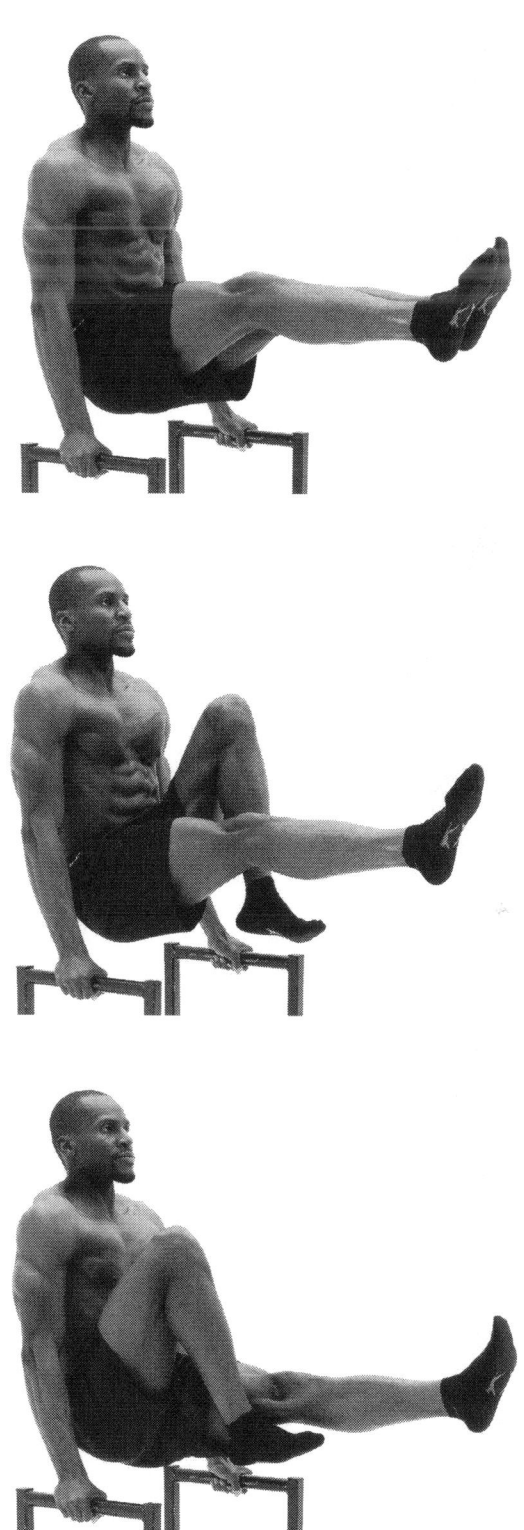

"Champions aren't made in gyms. Champions are made from something they have deep inside them — a desire, a dream, a vision. They have to have last-minute stamina, they have to be a little faster, they have to have the skill and the will. But the will must be stronger than the skill."

Muhammad Ali

6. Cardio & Conditioning

Welcome to HELL! Your final task is to power through the fire and come out the other side keeled over, dripping in sweat, but completely and utterly satisfied that you left absolutely NOTHING on the table.

Yes, this is a book focused on calisthenics, but it would be criminal to omit cardiovascular exercise and general conditioning, as this is the gateway to a truly SUPERHUMAN body. By performing these exercises you will condition your body to be able to work harder and go longer, thereby allowing you to compound your results exponentially.

You will also turn your body into a fat burning furnace, blasting belly fat and allowing your finely tuned muscles to come to the fore. For building popping six-pack abs and obliques in particular, this is non-negotiable. We are truly into no pain, no gain territory!

Remember, the name of the game here is not slow and steady; conditioning is all about intensity. Throw everything you have at the following exercises – if your heart isn't pounding, if you're not covered in sweat, then you're not training hard enough!

Don't be one of those people who sits idly on a bike, scrolling through their Facebook feed and working out their thumbs more than the rest of their body. And you better not skip it altogether either, because this guide comes as a package, just like your body.

If you're still in doubt as to the benefits of cardio and conditioning, here's a quick recap:

1. INCREASE METABOLISM: This becomes increasingly important as the years go by and your metabolism slows down. In order to achieve a peak state of being, use cardio to keep your metabolism running at full throttle!

2. KEEP YOUR HEART HEALTHY: Your heart just so happens to be the muscle that runs the entire show, and cardiovascular exercise is how you give it a workout. Look after your ticker, and it will look after you!

3. IMPROVE RECOVERY TIME: A spot of cardio after a heavy session can reduce your DOMS (Delayed Onset of Muscle Soreness) and rush healing, oxygen rich blood to the muscle tissues. Translation: you can get back in the game quicker!

4. BURN FAT AND LOOK AWESOME: The simple fact of the matter is that you will never burn that stubborn fat and achieve your dream body without cardio. So, how about we just quit all this jibber jabber and knock it out of the park!

6. Cardio & Conditioning

INTERVAL SPRINTS

Welcome to the pinnacle of cardio and conditioning exercises. Sprinting will get your heart pounding and your muscles working overtime to deliver INSANE results.

Super important: We must say it, but it truly is super important. Please, never perform cardiovascular activity without having had a thorough physical. Better safe than sorry.

Perform: 5-10 sets of 10-15 second bursts.

1. Take up the traditional starting position for a sprint, ready to spring off from one foot. If you are on a treadmill or free running, prepare to increase the speed.

2. With a powerful burst, break into as fast a sprint as you possibly can and do not stop until you reach your target to complete 1 set.

3. Rest for 30 secs or so and then go again. In this case, jogging can be a form of rest!

NB: Going from zero to everything can be risky, so make double sure that you have properly warmed up before launching into this kind of activity.

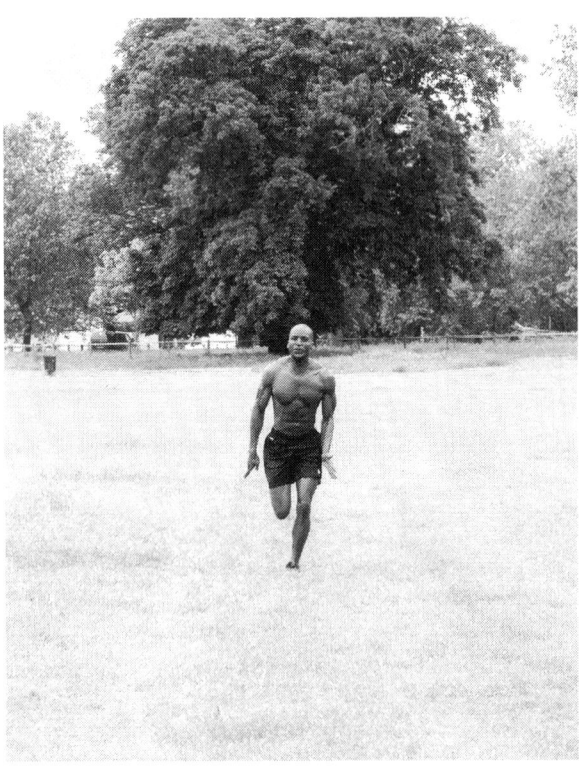
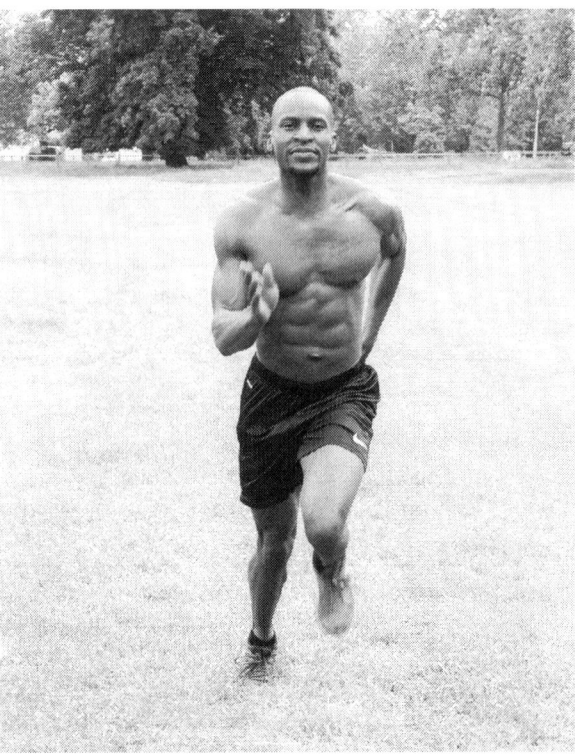

SKIPPING

Skipping is a great cardiovascular exercise that is often used for warming up or down as well as general fitness training.

Perform: 3-4 sets of 20-30 second bursts.

1. Grab your rope and swing it over your head.

2. From here you can either choose to jump both feet over the rope, or skip one foot at a time. If you're feeling really fancy, you can even do a criss cross.

Variation: Pick up a weighted rope for a greater challenge.

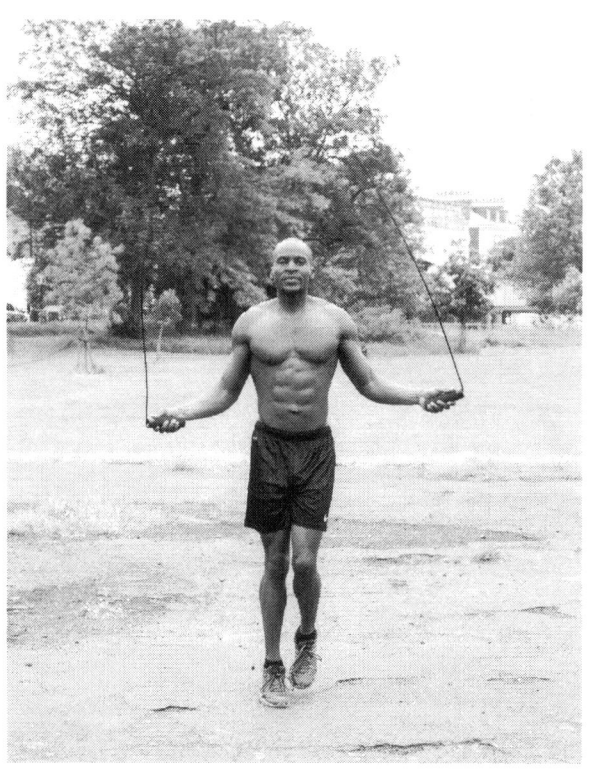 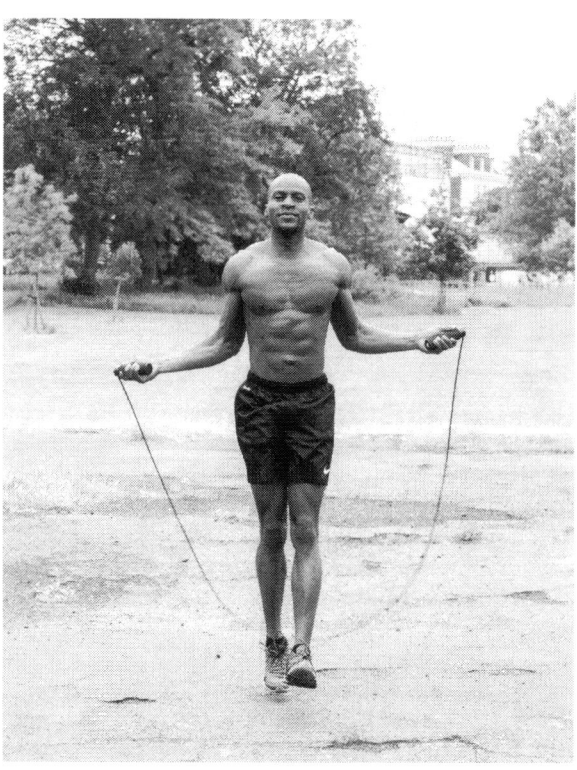

6. Cardio & Conditioning

JUMPING SQUAT

We covered the squat earlier on so you should be used to performing this movement in some capacity already, but it's now time to explore a more intense alternative.

Perform: 3-4 sets of 20-30 reps.

1. Take up the same starting position as regular squats, standing with your feet shoulder width apart.

2. Squat down as you would for regular squats.

3. Launch yourself into the air as high as possible.

4. Upon landing, bend your knees to absorb the impact and compete one rep, using the momentum generated to launch straight into the next rep.

Remember: You can always mix things up by working out against the clock instead of using a sets and reps system.

A mixture of the two, i.e. seeing how may reps you can perform in a certain amount of time, can be particularly effective when training cardio.

It's useful to have a training buddy when it comes to this kind of exercise, as it is pretty darn exhausting and you might find their support helps you find the strength to rock out that final rep.

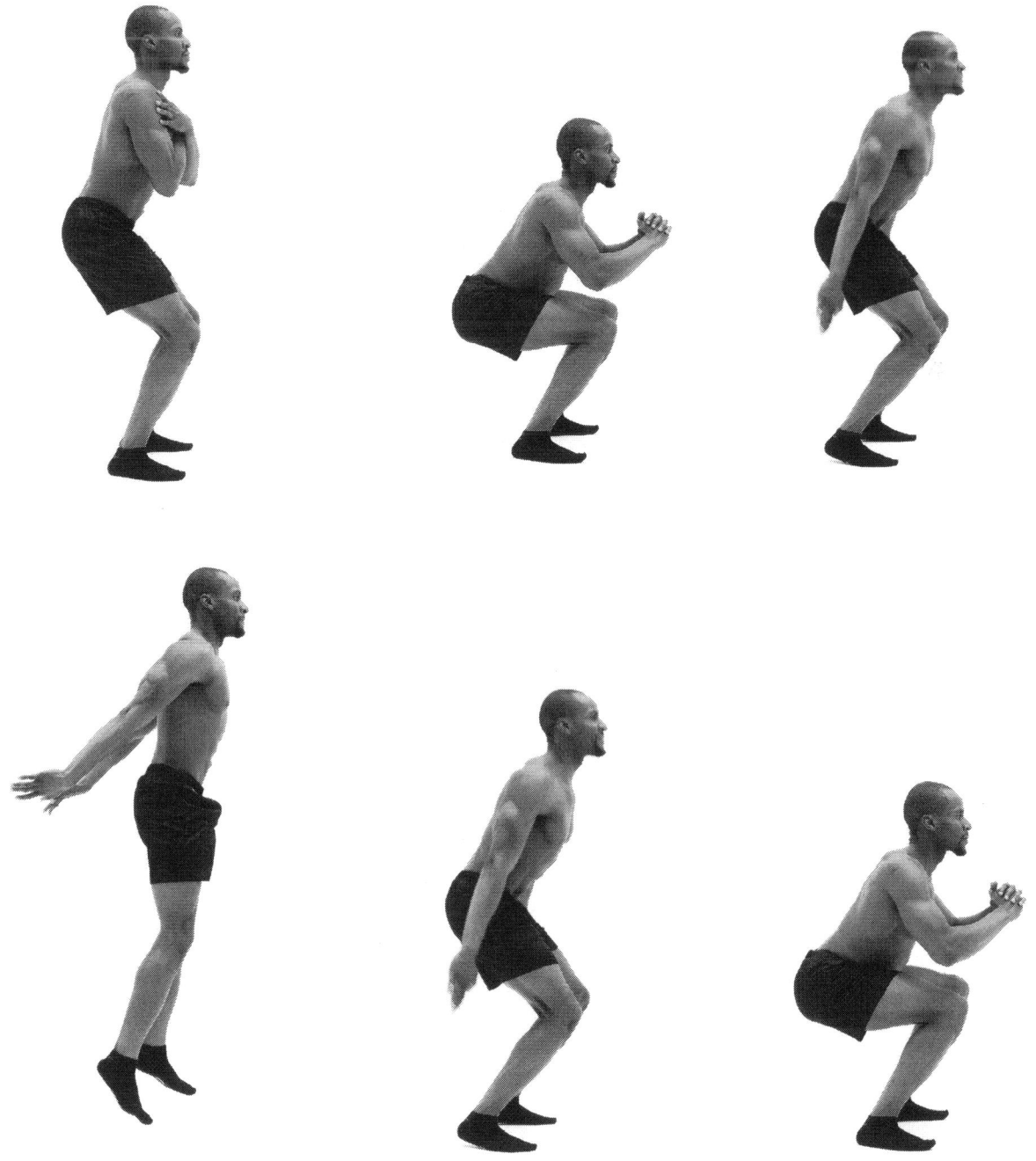

6. Cardio & Conditioning

SQUAT THRUST

We're getting a little more advanced now, but most people should still be comfortable with this exercise, with a little practice.

You'll soon notice that you are also getting a pretty decent full body workout in addition to your cardio hit. Embrace it. It's all part of become your best self.

Perform: 3-4 sets of 20-30 reps.

1. Squat down on your toes with your knees tucked against your chest and palms flat on floor in front of your feet.

2. Keeping your palms rooted, spring your feet off the ground and propel them backwards so you effectively land in the push-up position.

3. Reverse the movement, springing your feet back into the starting position to complete one repetition.

NB: If you've just performed this exercise for the first time, you will realize that it's more than just a cardio hit.

The squat thrust also calls upon your arms for support, your lower body for that explosive push off, and above all your core for hauling yourself into position.

For those who straight up hate cardio, there is at least some solace to be had in the knowledge that you are working hard on those other key areas, too!

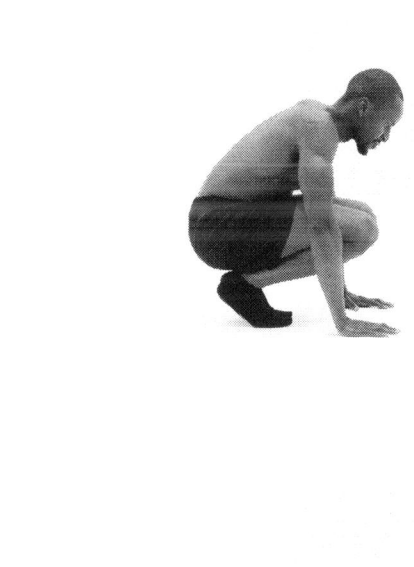
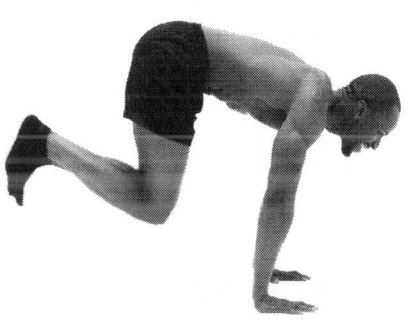
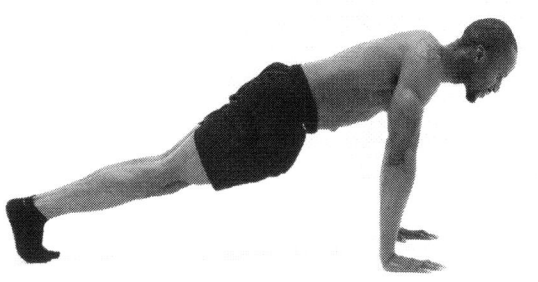
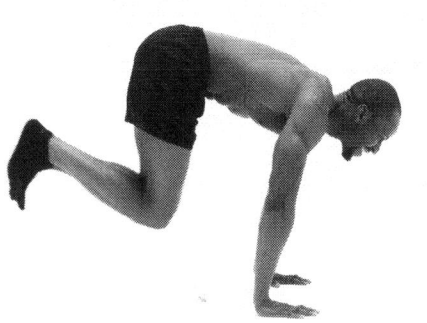
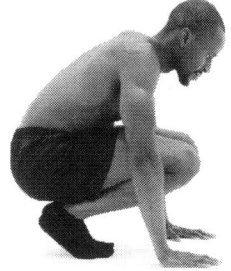

Mountain Climbers

Essentially a variation on the squat thrust, the mountain climber is an excellent addition to your cardio and conditioning repertoire.

Perform: 3-4 sets of 20-30 reps.

1. Take up the push-up position, except this time bring one foot right up until it's just behind your hands.

2. Spring your feet into the air and switch their positions, bringing the front one to the back and vice versa.

3. Reverse the action to bring your legs back to starting position to complete one rep. You can fire straight into the next rep from here.

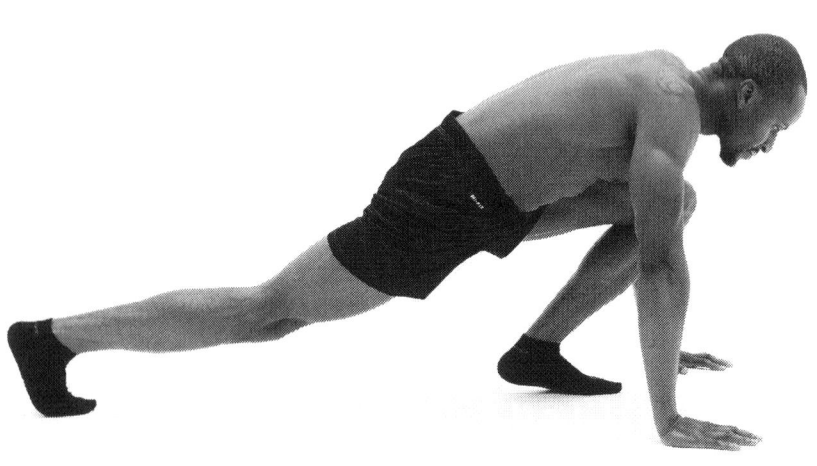

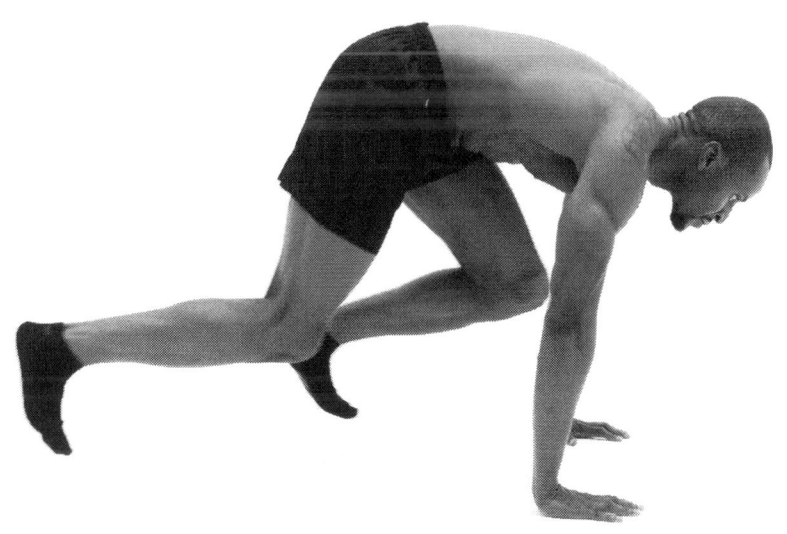

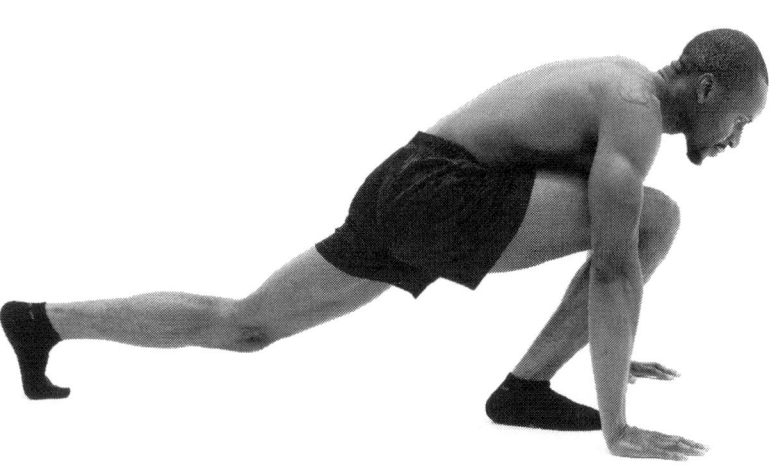

6. Cardio & Conditioning

JUMPING LUNGE

Another variation on an exercise we've already covered, the jumping lunge is a great way to condition your lower body at the same time as getting an intense cardio hit.

Perform: 3-4 sets of 6-10 reps on each leg.

1. Take up the lunge position with one foot forward and both knees bent, the rear one close to the ground.

2. Jump into the air, aiming to get as much height as possible, and switch leg positions, bringing the front one to the back and vice versa.

3. Bend your knees upon landing to complete one repetition and use the momentum generated to go on and perform a full set.

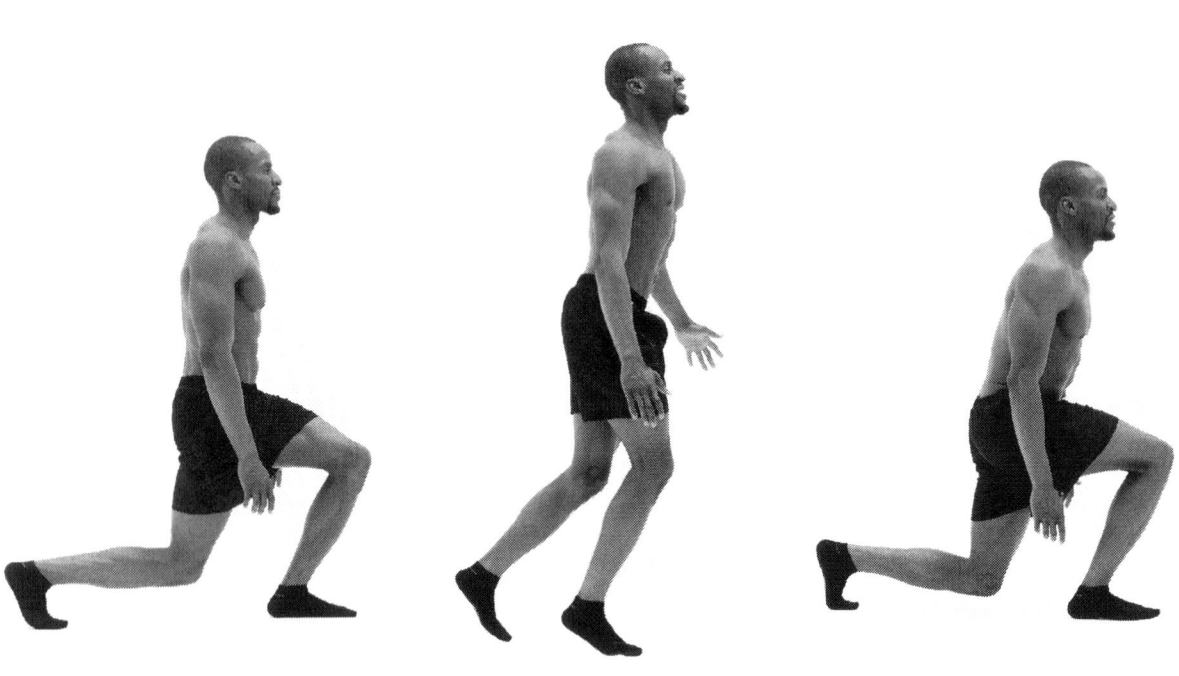

STAR JUMPS

Favored for its simplicity and famed for its effectiveness, the humble star jump is the staple of fitness regimes the world over. It is extremely likely that you have done this exercise before, but here's a reminder of how to complete it with proper form anyway.

Perform: 3-4 sets of 20-30 reps.

1. Stand up straight, feet together and arms by your sides.

2. Jump into the air stretching your arms and feet out to the sides.

3. Land with your feet wide apart and arms raised straight above your head.

4. Return to starting position by jumping up into the air again, bringing your feet back together and arms to your sides. You have now performed one repetition.

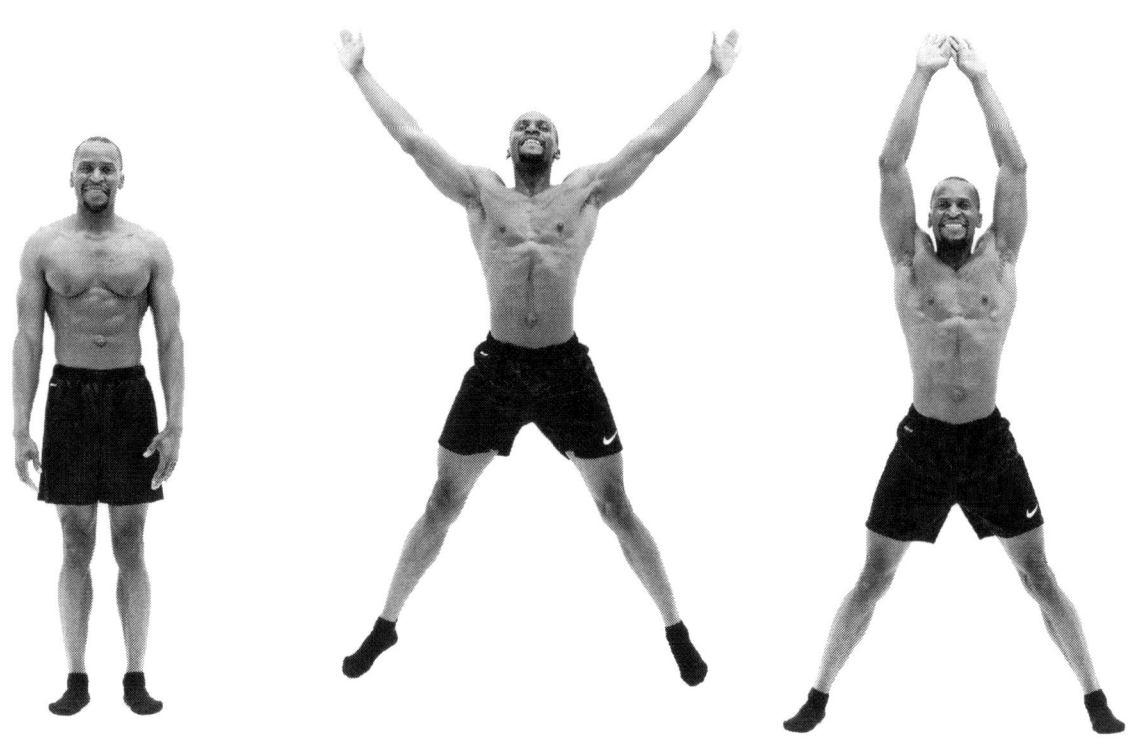

6. Cardio & Conditioning

BURPEES

You are about to call upon every muscle sinew in your body to complete one of the most effective conditioning exercises known to man, so get warmed up and prepare for pain!

Perform: 3-4 sets of 10-20 reps.

1. Take up the squat thrust position, crouched down on your toes with your knees tucked against your chest and palms flat on floor in front of your feet.

2. Palms rooted, spring your feet into the air and thrust your legs backwards so you land in the push-up position.

3. Reverse this movement, springing your feet into the air again and landing back in the starting position.

4. Jump straight upwards as high as you can, bending your knees upon landing to again assume the position in step 1 to complete one rep.

Remember: Keep it moving with exercises like this. Pushing on through exhaustion is how progress is made. Never just go through the motions or quit as soon as the going gets tough!

You may find it particularly difficult to keep track of sets and reps when your heart is busy pumping oxygen to every extremity, so setting a timer and working to the clock is a great way to train if you're going solo.

If you have a training partner, have them count you down, and don't be afraid of a little competition. You might just bring the best out of each other.

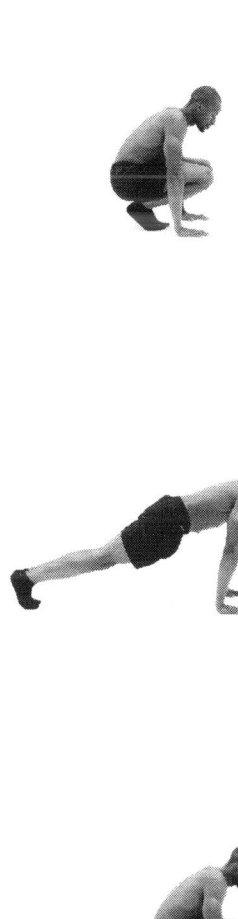
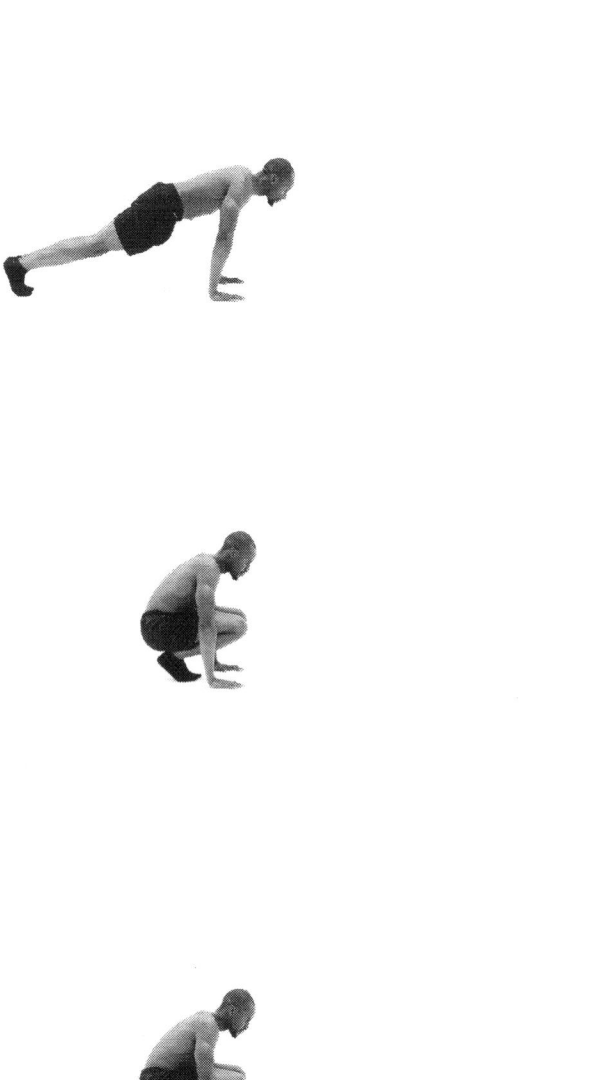
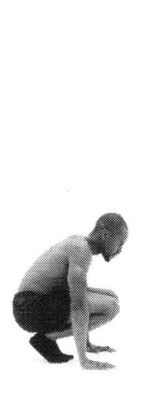

6. Cardio & Conditioning

ADVANCED BURPEES

Essentially the same as the burpee, except we're tossing a push-up into the middle of each rep. Some call it the 'bastard', and you're about to find out why!

Perform: 3-4 sets of 10-20 reps.

1. Assume the same starting position as the burpee, crouched down, knees just behind your hands, braced for the punishment to come.

2. Now kick your feet back to push-up position as before.

3. Knock out 1 push-up.

4. When you are back at the top of the push-up position, kick your feet back to the crouched position.

5. Now jump straight up into the air, aiming for the moon!

6. Land back in the crouched position and go again.

Are you feeling the burn? If you said no, you're lying. But fear not, for we are about to draw this cardio and conditioning section to a close.

We have one more offering which is sure to attract some double takes out in public, but don't be afraid to go all in. After all, you get out exactly what you put in.

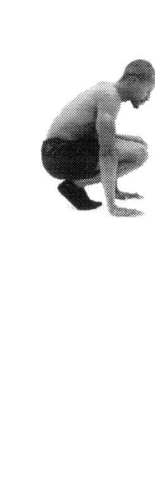 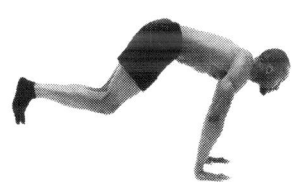 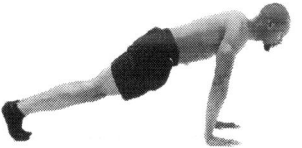

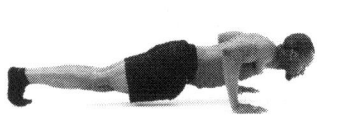 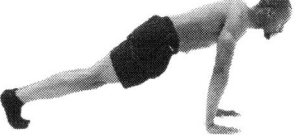 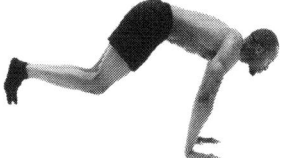

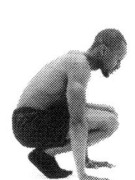 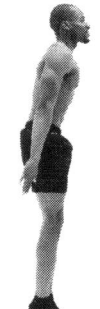 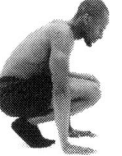

6. Cardio & Conditioning

BEAR CRAWLS

This is another brutal conditioning exercise, but pain really does mean gain here so commit to completing it and you will see and feel the benefits.

Perform: 3-4 sets of 15-20 second crawls.

1. Take up the push-up position.

2. Place one hand forward, and bring the opposite foot forward too. Continue crawling like this, alternating your hands and legs, until you reach your threshold.

3. Repeat for allocated number of sets.

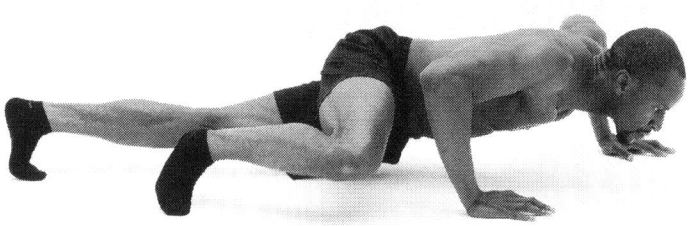

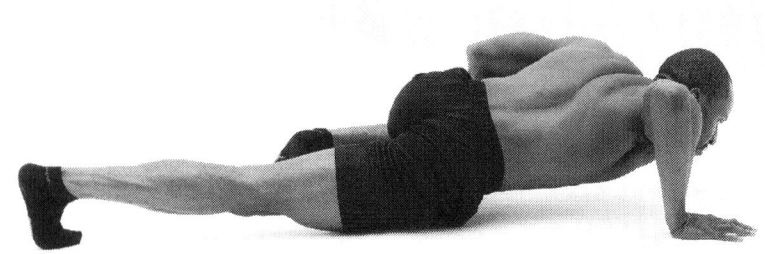

OTHER

You can probably see a trend building with cardio and conditioning – intense bursts of activity, followed by a short rest before going in all over again.

Cycling, rowing, boxing, circuits, swimming etc. are other great ways to get the blood pumping so don't be afraid to throw your own interests and hobbies into the mix.

It is generally recommended to perform 30-60 minutes of cardio per day. In addition to the benefits you already know of, you may also experience a myriad of other pros. These include reduced stress and anxiety, clarity of thought, improved sleep and even a potent antidote to depression. It really pays, then, to find a way to get your fix.

So long as your heart is pounding and your brow is dripping, you are doing cardio. It doesn't have to be by the book, but it does have to be done, and it does have to be tough. That is non-negotiable for those seeking SUPERHUMAN status.

Our mantra is simple: train hard. Two words that need to be etched into your mind whenever you enter the field of battle. Do not turn up to participate, turn up to WIN!

If you are training solo, every day should be an endeavor to reach a personal best or achieve something new. If you have a training buddy, push each other to higher levels by competing on every exercise. You will be shocked at just how far this takes you.

So, with that final gut-busting burst of activity we conclude this complete rundown of calisthenics exercises. You now possess the very same knowledge as the elite.

You have witnessed the unparalleled power of bodyweight exercise, and you have step-by-step instructions to achieve the body of your dreams.

Depending on your current level of ability, you may be ready to dive in at the deep end, or you might have to flip right back to the beginning and start at square one.

Our one key piece of advice is to understand and accept your level, and progress at your own pace. It is far more beneficial to make steady progress with proper form than it is to rush ahead and completely fail to achieve your objectives.

Flip the page for more advice on progressing with calisthenics.

7. Progressing With Calisthenics

Like any form of exercise it is essential to nail down the basics before progressing. In fact, the same is true of anything in life. As the old saying goes, walk before you can run!

You might be tempted to dive straight into a handstand or attempt a human flag but without sufficient practice you will not possess the strength or technique required in order to perform more advanced exercises.

Before you attempt something new, ask yourself one simple question and commit to answering truthfully: 'have I completed each number of sets or the hold time allocated for the easier exercises in this book absolutely perfectly?'

If the answer is 'no', then revisit the areas you still need to work on. By doing this you will gradually build a body that is properly prepared for advanced bodyweight exercises.

To help you reach that level in the fastest possible time, we've put together a beginner's calisthenics routine for you absolutely free. See the next page to get your copy now.

Once you have surpassed the beginner's level, or if you are already at intermediate or advanced capability, there is still plenty of room for improvement.

Arguably the greatest thing about calisthenics is that the possibilities are almost endless when it comes to inventing variations on established exercises, which means progress never stops, unless you do!

Once you can perform a base exercise, and have mastered each variation thereof, feel free to experiment with your own interpretations. So long as you maintain proper form, you will continue to experience phenomenal growth.

It is at this stage, when you are mastering high level exercises and coming up with your own innovative variations, that you can truly claim SUPERHUMAN status! To get there faster, join us at purecalisthenics.com for more resources.

You can also find the rest of the books in this series by searching 'Pure Calisthenics' on Amazon. In the meantime, get on a training program and go hard!

See you at SUPERHUMAN!

The Pure Calisthenics Team

8. BONUS: FREE TRAINING PROGRAM

You've got the exercises, now get the program! Download your bodyweight training routine free now and get on the road to total body perfection.

Here at Pure Calisthenics we're all about progressive teaching, and that is exactly what this program has been designed to achieve.

Build a solid foundation with this fundamental calisthenics routine, broken down into a full week of exercises, complete with suggested sets and reps.

Don't leave your results to chance; follow a proven program and take your first steps on the road to SUPERHUMAN right now!

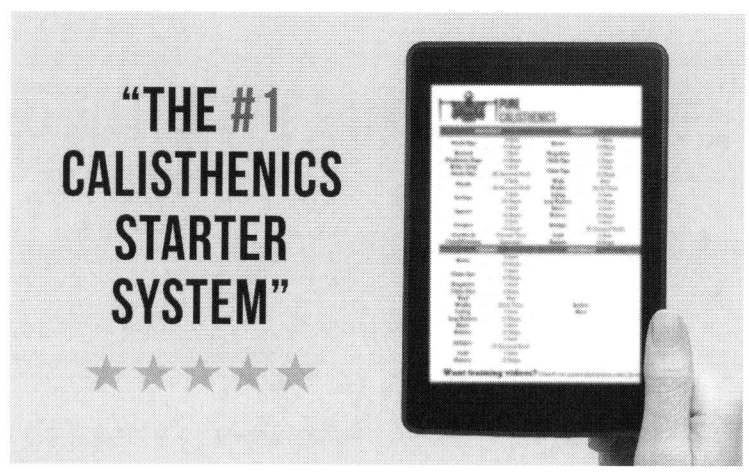

Visit www.purecalisthenics.com for your free program!

LIKE THIS BOOK?

The calisthenics community is all about sharing ideas and growing together. With that in mind, here's a few ways you can get involved:

1. If you got value from this book, or the free bonus training program, we'd be super stoked if you could head on over to your Amazon purchase history to leave a review.

2. The most powerful way to boost your progress is to share your journey with a friend. Put a call out on Facebook and Twitter, share this guide with a training partner and go crush it together!

3. To see our other books and resources, search 'Pure Calisthenics' on Amazon and visit www.purecalisthenics.com for bodyweight training tips, equipment reviews, nutrition advice and more!

So, all that remains to say is thanks for picking up this book. Don't forget to grab your free program and, as always, train hard!

The Pure Calisthenics Team

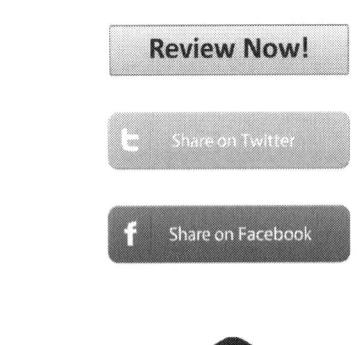

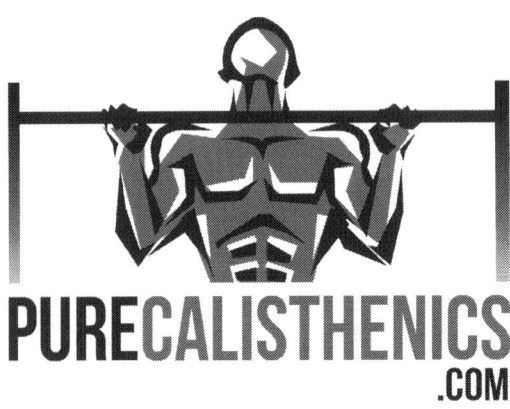

Printed in Great Britain
by Amazon